The Three Mystics

of Celtic Reiki

By
Martyn Pentecost

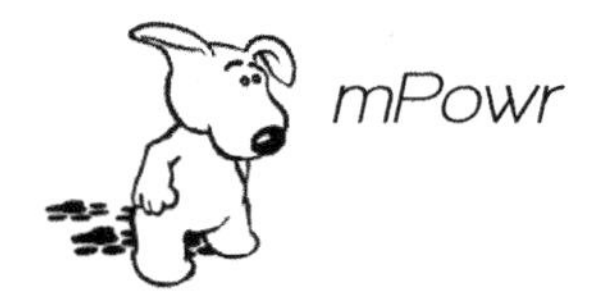

First Published in Great Britain 2010 by mPowr (Publishing) Limited
www.mpowrpublishing.com
www.celtic-reiki.com

A catalogue record for this book is available from the British Library
ISBN – 978-1-907282-40-9

Cover Design by Martyn Pentecost
mPowr Publishing 'Clumpy™' Logo by e-nimation.com
Clumpy™ and the Clumpy™ Logo are trademarks of mPowr Limited

Made by Book Brownies!

Books published by mPowr Publishing are made by Book Brownies. A Book Brownie is about so high, with little green boots, a potato-like face and big brown eyes. These helpful little creatures tenderly create every book with kindness, care and a little bit of magic! Before shipping, a Book Brownie will jump into the pages—usually at the most gripping chapter or a part that pays particular attention to food—and stay with that book, always. This means that every mPowr Publishing book comes with added enchantment (and occasional chocolate smudges!) so that you get a warm, fuzzy feeling of love with the turn of every page!

The arts of compassion, strength, and wisdom await you...

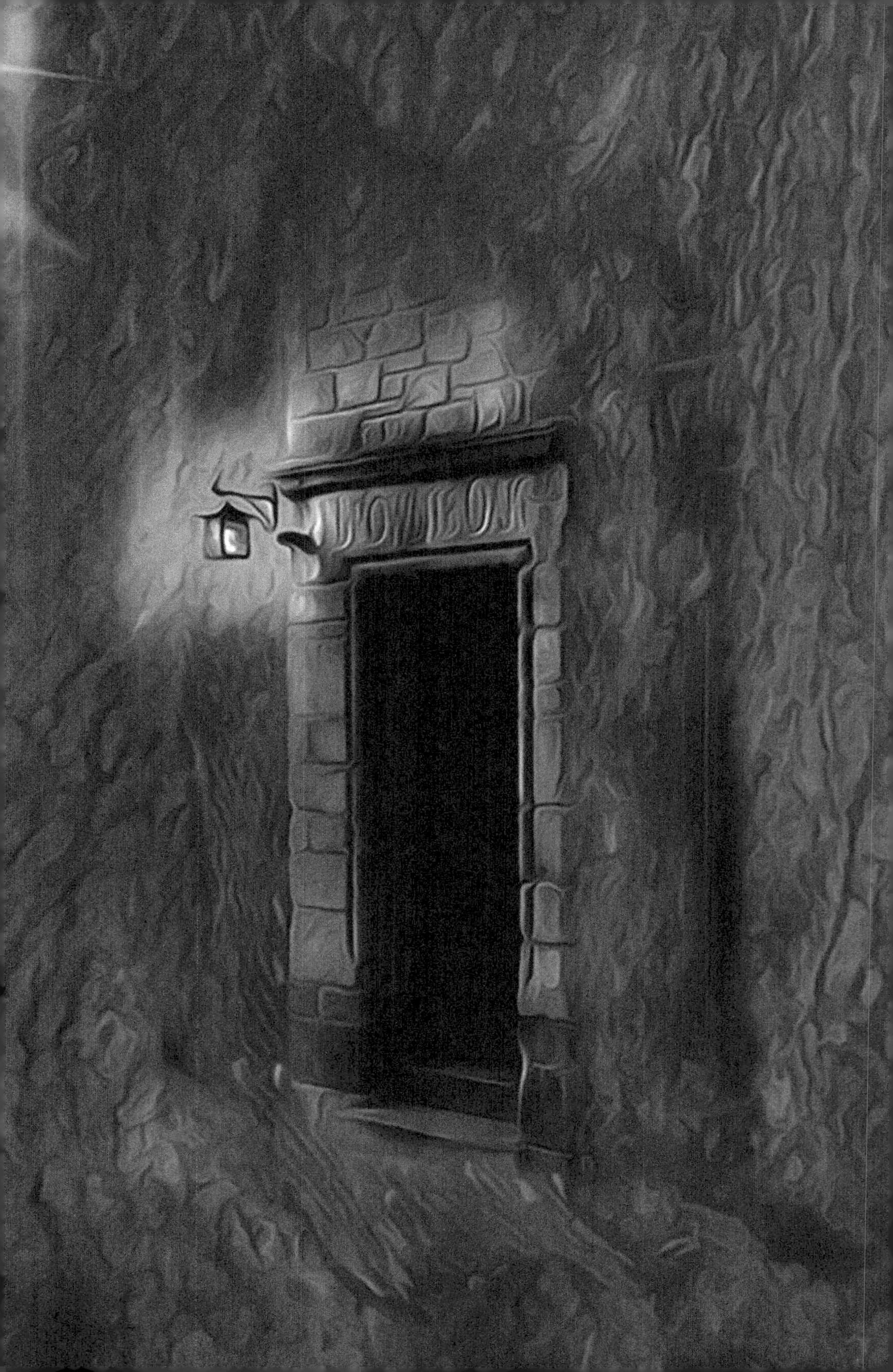

Contents

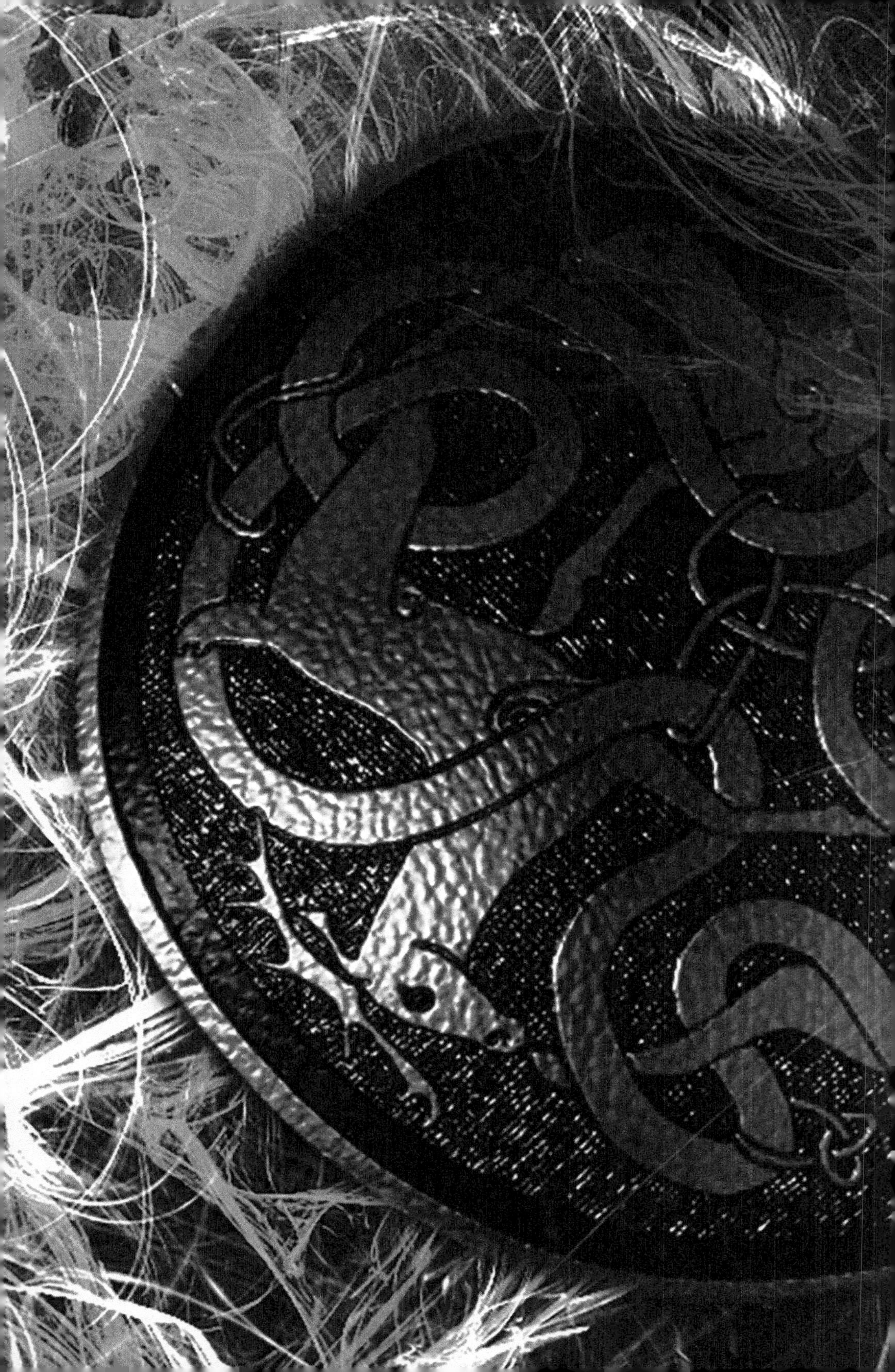

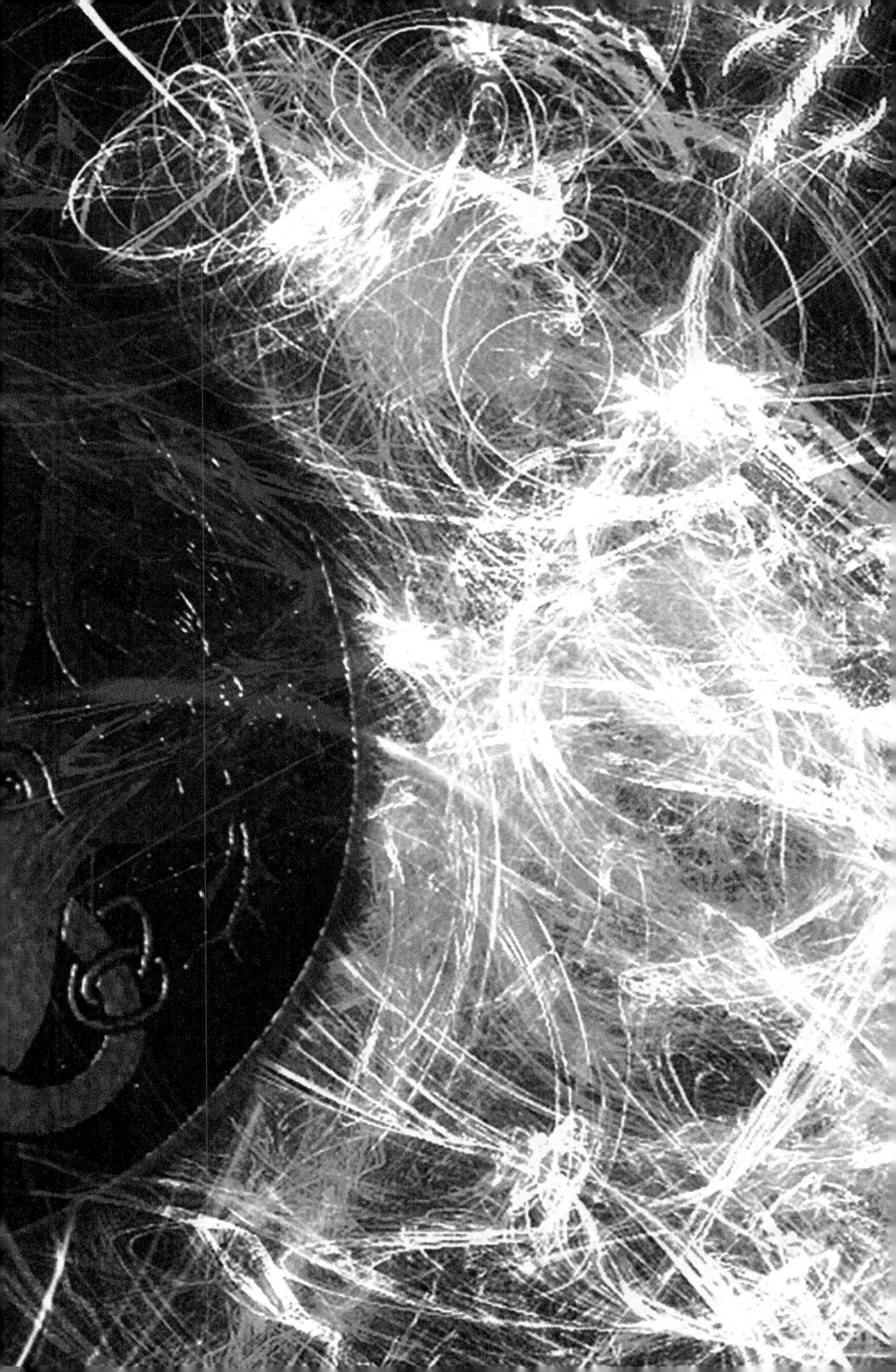

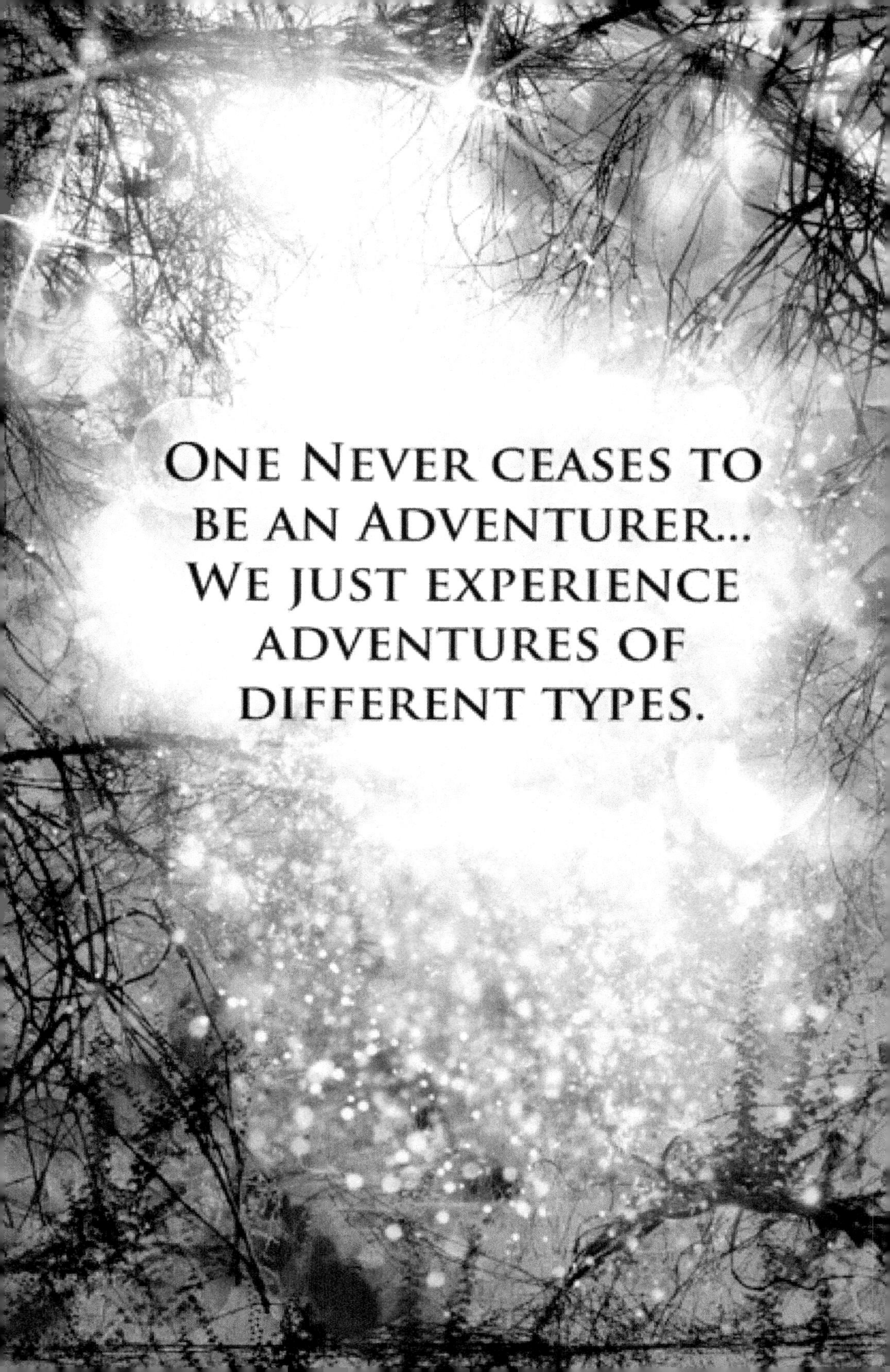
One Never ceases to
be an Adventurer...
We just experience
adventures of
different types.

THE ADVENTURE CONTINUES...

The exploration of Celtic Reiki is unusual in many ways, none more so than the recognition of a profound paradox in the study of the practice and mastery of our art. In the Adventurer's Guide, we investigated the use of Avatar State to connect with and envelop the attitude of the five Mystics of Celtic Reiki. In this book, we shall continue this voyage by examining and working with the three mystics of practitionership. However, as you are studying these mystics, defining them from your own viewpoint, learning how to integrate their ways with your own, it will soon become apparent that you are doing so as the Adventurer!

Therefore, it is not until you are practicing, that you truly represent the three mystics. In other words, what is to follow is the Adventurer assisting you in the theory of practice; a theory that will help you to achieve practitioner status. So, all the way through your Home Experience, through the practice sessions and even during the elements of mastery, you will be walking in the Adventurer's shoes.

The very point at which you work in Avatar State to connect to the Wise One (for example), not to learn, but to treat a person professionally for the first time, will be a completely different experience. It is at that point you are no longer intending to learn, but to support your client's healing processes and it is this scenario that creates the vital difference between the Adventurer and the Wise One (or the other Mystics).

Yet, even then, the Adventurer is present; watching, absorbing, learning new things that will improve the results and offer a richer depth of experience. This may at first seem a little lacklustre, especially if you are eager to experience the Mystics that exist beyond the Adventurer perspective. Nevertheless, it is this very paradox that will present you with one of the most profound aspects of your learning.

There are three distinct 'methods' of reading this book (and the Master's Companion): as an Adventurer when studying; as a practitioner Mystic when reconciling results and feedback from treatments; or as the Master Mystic, preparing to teach Celtic Reiki Mastery to others. You could read this book a hundred times, cover to cover, whilst studying; you could know every line, word for word, and yet, the very first time you read as a practitioner Mystic, it will be like reading a completely different book!

It will be as if somebody came along and erased all the pages, typing a whole new set. Entire passages will appear from nowhere and there will be various concepts, philosophies, and techniques that you have never actually seen before. This is, in a psychological perspective, due to the way our brains work. When learning, we filter out anything that does not help us learn, but as soon as you begin to practice professionally, situations and circumstances will arise that become very relevant. This newfound relevance will shift your focus to recognise and consciously grasp what was previously filtered out.

So, during your reading as an Adventurer, you are more likely to perceive what will help you learn. As the practitioner Mystics, your perception will change to glean practical information from the book (and online content). And, when you read these words as a Master, your focus will be on helping your students to learn as best they can.

Another truly remarkable outcome from this filtering process is that, no matter how confused you are at first, there will come a time where everything just clicks into place. You will completely comprehend every aspect of your art, as if it were the most natural thing in the world; something you have always known (which of course, you have!).

Even though on your first reading of this book, you will be doing so as an Adventurer Mystic, it would soon become confusing if that differentiation was made throughout, so what follows refers to the Mystics as they will be during your practitionership (and mastery) rather than the effects of Avatar State during your study and apprenticeship.

The practitionership is multifaceted and moves beyond the traditional view of what the term 'practitioner' means, both in the sense of Reiki practice and in the wider scope of complementary therapy. The Celtic Reiki system is a personal development practice (Adventurer's Guide p.19) that combines many different methods to expose aspects of 'therapy' that are very often misinterpreted or missed out altogether.

The standard perception of therapies and their training is; the practitioner heals themselves and then goes on to heal others. This creates the notion of two distinct processes - rather like oil and water. The upshot of this is often the embedding of 'implicit rules' that are detrimental to the therapeutic processes of any treatment. For example: the belief that a practitioner needs to be completely healed and 'perfect' before they treat others; the practitioner requires no therapy once they have begun to practice and if the need for therapy arises, they should stop treating others; that our learning and need for developments is finite and 'ends' at some point.

What is even more pernicious is the duality that these implicit beliefs create - the concept of 'their stuff', 'my energy', 'my energy taking on board their stuff'. Of course there is a need for practitioners to act professionally, to remained focused on their clients, and to cope with the situations they encounter. However, the therapist that perceives treatment as being simultaneously beneficial to client and practitioner learns how to cope with (and actively transform) the dis-eases and challenges that arise.

When the implicit rules of duality ('me' and 'them', 'mine' and 'theirs') become the explicit Lores of Celtic Reiki ('we are one, separated by illusion and striving for wholeness'), an amazing synthesis develops and suddenly the isolation of dis-ease melts away to the light of unity. It is this illusion of separateness that historically formed the dual approach to treatment and everyday perception of the world, yet our intellectual understanding of 'oneness' and interconnectivity, enables us to use duality in a very different way.

By segmenting our practitionership into three contrasting definitions, one externally-facing, one internally-focused, and one that alternates between the other two, we create a practitionership that leads us to true mastery. Mastery, not of the self or of others, but mastery of unity and wholeness. This trinity of what we know as Mystics, are defined by perspective, rather than separation.

This is a feature of Celtic Reiki that is most apparent in the Mountain Range, where the Northern Peaks represent oneness viewed from multiple perspectives and the Volcanic South is indicative of separation and the making of autonomous 'entities'. In other words - the Northern Peaks are a single range of mountains that can be viewed from the summits or the foothills, whereas the Volcanoes of the South create shapes that seem to be separate from the world around them.

The three Mystics of Celtic Reiki are not three distinct and isolated 'beings'; they are one entity, viewed from three alternate perspectives. This entity is the Practitioner, but more than that, it exists at the point where the Adventurer (Student/ Apprentice) is combined with the Master (Teacher/Harvester) to form an eternal and infinite dynamic: the question and the answer; the observer and the observed; the naivety and the knowing; to know all there is to know, except what it is not to know.

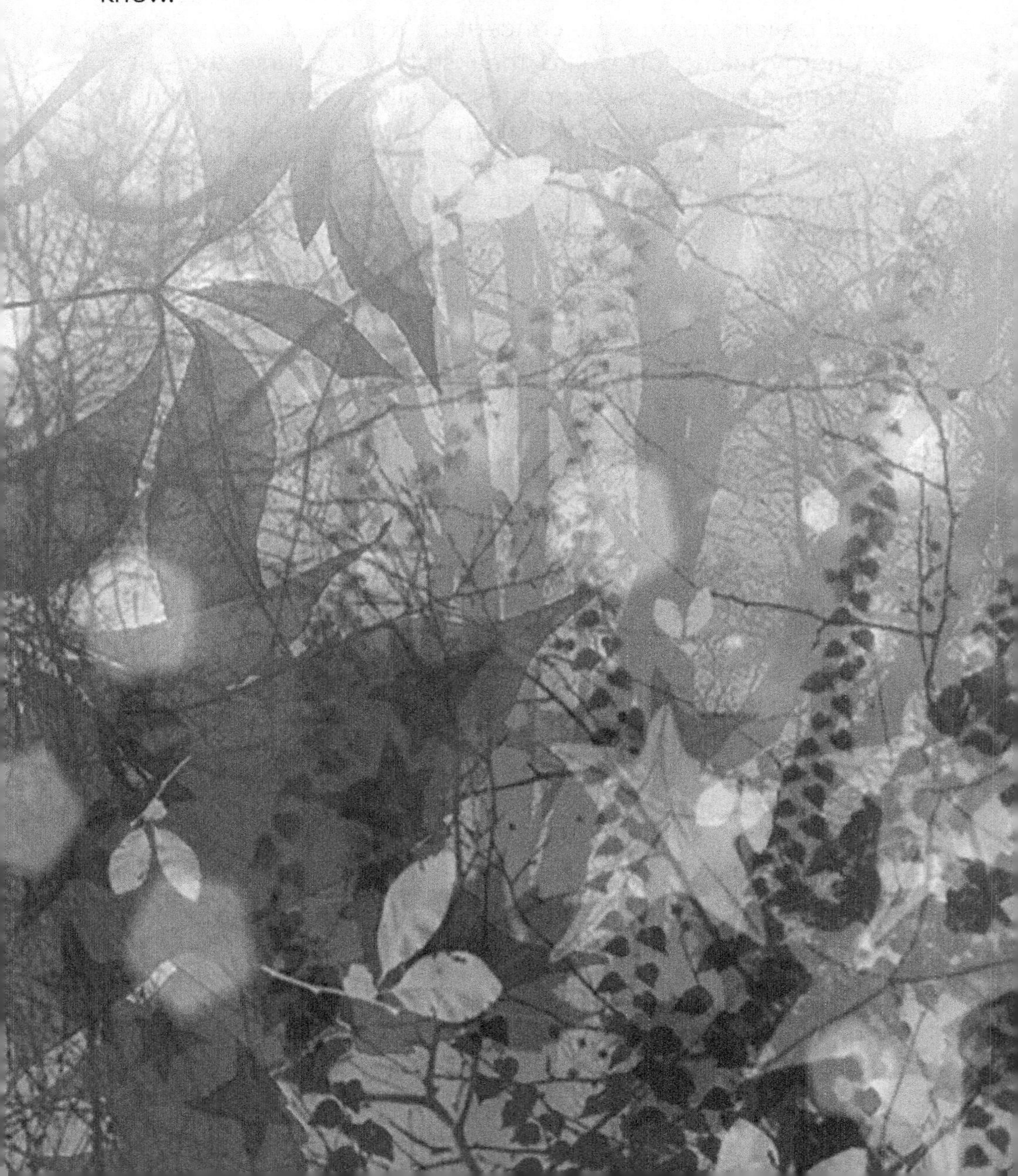

The Three Mystical arts of Practitionership

The Practitionership of Celtic Reiki has three strands that are derived from the Adventurer Mystic and converge, at an advanced level, to form the Master Mystic. Each strand enables the Celtic Reiki Apprentice to specialise and focus on the diverse elements of our practice, whilst offering the Master a means of consolidating the intricate nuances of each art into one, 'smooth' Personal Development methodology.

The three strands are each represented by a Mystic that is connected to via Avatar State and worked with to learn, use, and adapt the different practices that form facets of the Celtic Reiki whole. Each Mystic represents a perspective, rather like that of an essence, however this perspective has a deeper integration with the behaviour and attitude of the Practitioner. An essence will affect the user and focus of any practice, the Mystic is embodied by the Practitioner and, as a result, both Practitioner and Mystic are completely altered by the relationship.

We could use the analogy of a house to understand the different elements of Celtic Reiki: the Mystics, the Lores and the Realms. If Celtic Reiki was your home, then every room could be represented by a Realm - these are places, not necessarily physical spaces, but a concept of each, individual room (you could use a physical space as a study or bedroom, but still have a clear idea of what purposes these are used for).

Therefore, the Woodland Realm has a purpose, in which various actions are completed. The Standing Stones, has a different purpose and even though there is a certain amount of overlap in the actions that are conducted in this Realm, the context of the actual Realm, completely changes the results. (Imagine reading in bed and reading in the study; how does this change the mental image you have?)

In this scenario, one might assume the Mystics are the people that live in the house, although it is more accurate to view the relationships between people as representative of the Mystics. For example, one person could be a mother, daughter, aunt, sister, wife, and niece. In a wider context, she could also be a friend, acquaintance, manager, employer, employee, consultant, teacher, mentor, therapist, idol, icon, and so on. The point is that this one person has many roles that are contrasting in definition. Her behaviour when she is in the position of an employer would be different than when she is being a wife. She will act differently to her children than towards her 'fans'. Interacting as a daughter will probably cause her to feel vary different than when in the company of friends. The Adventurer Mystic would act very differently to the prospect of treating another person, than the Wise One - one would be exploring and learning, whilst the other would focus on the client's needs and the attainment of conducive results.

Hence, the Mystics are relationships, personas and defined characters that we embody to such an extent it actually changes our behaviour, actions and results.

Lores are the ways of doing things in the house; so some will be 'loose' dynamics, such as: we clean up after ourselves. Others would be more rigid: We place the recycling out for collection on a Tuesday night after 8pm. Once again, the Lore is not the physical act, it is the concept of the act, meaning that a rigid action would be of EarthLore, whereas an action that has no defined structure could be EnergyLore. (The dynamics that have no definition, but still affect the household would be CosmicLore.)

In other words, Realms define the tools and practices of Celtic Reiki, Lores are the 'way' in which we conduct our mastery and Mystics create the relationships we have in our practices - with Celtic Reiki, our clients, our students and ourselves.

The Mystics of the Practitionership provide an opportunity to diversify and really hone in on the different aspects of practice by placing an emphasis on different perspectives. The first Mystic we encounter - the Wise One - is orientated towards other people, although she can also help us to face inwards for self-healing. Her sphere of influence is rooted in healing, worldly knowledge and evolution.

The Warrior gazes into the self and the depths of wisdom we hold inside of ourselves, as well as bringing hidden qualities to the surface. Like the Wise One, he can direct his attention to the outer world, for the purpose of prophecy, teaching and proactive defence. Whereas the Wise One is usually motivated by DarkLore (inside become outside), the Warrior forms an

Avatar that brings the outside into the inner world (EnergyLore). The Wise One is accustomed to take what is hidden within the self and places it in others for us to treat and heal with an 'external focus'. The Warrior, however, knows that everything is a reflection of what exists within us, so focuses on strengthening the self.

This realisation helps us to grasp two different perspectives of the same foundation to happiness. One perspective sees some form of dis-ease that hinders or even prevents happiness from being experienced. The other views happiness as obtainable through the proactive and positive growth of the self. The Warrior takes responsibility for the creation of happiness and wellbeing, whilst the Wise One hones in on the elements that block happiness for others (and ultimately the self).

The Alchemist appears to have one eye on the self and another on the outside world, though in actuality, he shifts his gaze from one to the other so quickly as to be unnoticeable. He knows our inner desires and wants, he is also worldly-wise inasmuch as he knows how things 'work'. Using a combination of emotional wanting and solid-world definition, he creates wholeness and fulfilment. Therefore, the Alchemist is the Mystic of manifestation, success and prosperity.

To truly understand the Mystics, one must have a clear definition of each Mystic and then completely blur the lines between them, so they merge into each other. The Practitioner degree of Celtic Reiki is the definition part of the process, where we form strong and lasting philosophies about each individual Mystic.

To illustrate this, let us briefly examine how each Mystic functions from the perspective of holistic layering, using the four definitions: spiritual, cerebral, emotional, and physical. Here we see that there are some initial Lores that will help define our Mystics.

- Each Mystic influences all four layers
- Every Mystic acts of all four layers
- The three Mystics are physically orientated, whilst being centred upon their own specific layer: Wise One/ spiritual, Warrior/emotional, Alchemist/cerebral.
- It is only their appearance that offers the illusion of

having separate methodologies, for the purpose of all the Mystics is identical.

So, from these Lores, we understand that the Wise-One is spiritually centred, whilst focusing on the physical world results. When they act, they do so on all layers. However, their actions only present the illusion of being different from the Warrior and Alchemist, for their actual goal is the same.

Before we investigate how each Mystic achieves this single aim, let us explore further, the unique definitions of each Mystic in greater detail.

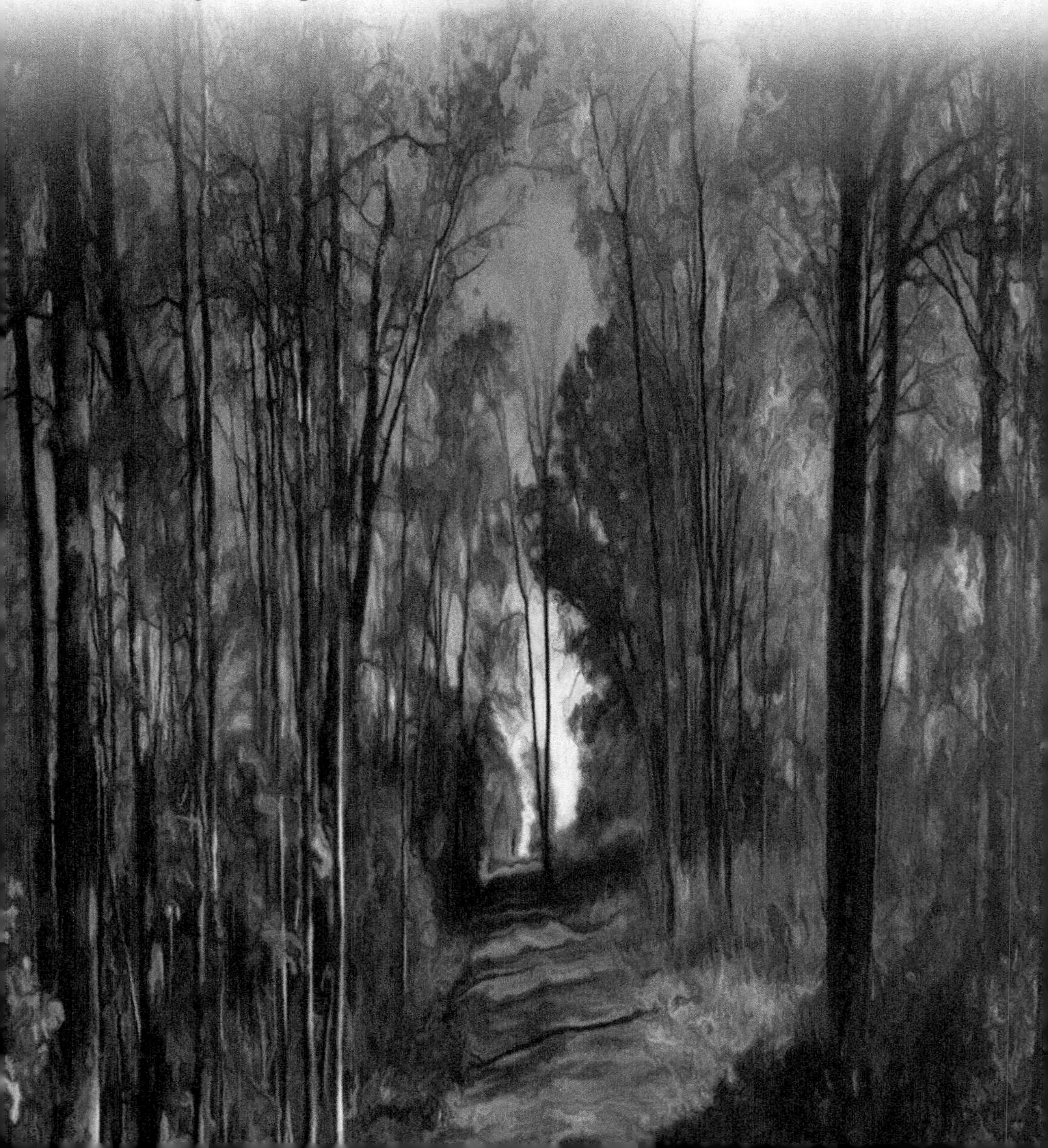

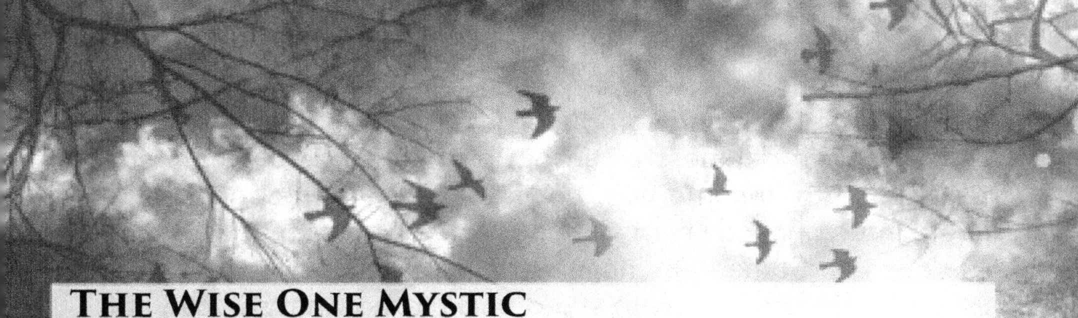

THE WISE ONE MYSTIC

She stood watching across the grocery store, saturated with the experience of the man who seemed so beyond sadness as to be tragic in demeanour. She could see right into him, not with her eyes, but with an inner-vision; a knowing. Underneath the simple appearance of a man conducting his weekly shop, was a darkness, a pain that hinted at a person who felt himself irredeemable. In every way, this man was lost.

She hesitated; wanting so much to help, but knowing that it must be his choice to begin the process of healing. So, she just stood for a while, pretending to check oranges for freshness, whilst enveloping the physical environment with essences. Of course, she knew that for him to get any benefit, she must move herself closer to his perspective. If she could find his way of looking at the world, she could alter the essences to exist in his perception. The mere recognition of an essence would spark some form of healing.

So she searched herself, to find some common ground; some vague connection between them. When she thought of how she was once broken hearted, he jolted, as if pulled upward and back by his shoulders.

"Has your heart been broken?" She asked introspectively.

Feeling a wave of empathy wash over her, she began to fill her thoughts with Quert, Tinne, Rose Quartz and Freja, knowing instinctively that these may help the man, if he could only notice some change, some internal expansion that lifted him from his despair.

For a moment he caught her eye, looking straight at her, as if he knew she was attempting to help him. She smiled a gentle smile and thought, "If you need my help, all you need do is ask..."

A moment later, he was stepping across the aisle with a sense of purpose and began to come towards her... The Wise

One is empathic and intuitive, she knows others' pain and trauma, because she feels it within herself. This Mystic is not concerned about being completely healed or perfect, but about using her own darkness as an opportunity to help others and heal the Earth in some way. For the Wise One recognises the innate interconnectivity of all things; the oneness that we share.

Sometimes, her need to help can be overwhelming, although she knows how to stand back, to do what she can at a distance, and to wait until those who need help ask for it. This is not always a definite, verbal request, for it may come in a look, a feeling, or the mere acceptance of the essences the Wise One presents to them.

There are many subtleties in treatment, the sudden jolt of the shoulders, a pulling backwards, the twitch of a finger or eyelid. The Wise One is versed in all these minute clues to a person's receptivity to healing and their acknowledgement of connection to higher layers of being. Yet, she also knows that to create this connection, she needs to look inside herself, rather than out into the world. By recognising her own challenges, she discovers some resonant perspective with those she treats. It is this common theme that connects people, for without some shared experience or similar perception of the world, we simply pass each other by.

The Wise One is excellent at knowing which essences to use for different situations, not because one essence is right and another wrong, but simply because each perspective offers definition and structure to a treatment. She is also aware when essences can be adjusted and altered to achieve deeper, longer-lasting results.

Tip for the Adventurer

Connect every situation or circumstance you encounter with two or three essences and state explicitly to yourself why you have chosen these specifically. If you are in the habit of knowing how to connect essences with issues and why, you will find treatments and consultations much easier

CONNECTING TO THE WISE ONE

There is a deep sense of 'knowing' when you first connect to the Wise One Mystic, through Avatar State. This is imbued with both an indescribable compassion and the knowledge that everything is just as it should be. Over time, it is this feeling of serene perfection that remains as a lasting sensation, because the other aspects of compassion and knowing will become second nature to you.

This means that through professional practice, you become the Wise One, with all their facets and qualities seeming no different than how you feel now - the benevolence is so overwhelming that it will haunt you; always remaining as a reminder of something more, something greater.

As you transition from the Adventurer Mystic, the following technique will help you to connect fully to the Wise One and help you to gain an innate insight into the embodiment of this healing Mystic. There will be a distinct change between the sensations you consciously experience in the study of this technique and the connection to the Wise One in a 'live', professional situation.

As such, it is important that you use the technique throughout your training and until you are completely confident with your practice in the professional environment. Even if you feel completely comfortable and au fait with the Avatar State connection to the Wise One, failure to use the technique presented here, could mean that you carry-over the Adventurer perspective of the Wise One, even in a professional situation.

This is because the technique in itself is a step-by-step progression towards the Wise One Mystic that works in a uniform and consistent way. What does change over time is the sensation you will experience when conducting the routine.

The Master Mystic relies on these sensations alone to connect to the Wise One from the mastery perspective, and if you are using the same indicators that you experienced in a training environment, you will most likely achieve the same results.

Using this method as a learning tool and one that provides a consistent baseline (of result rather than experience) will offer you the 'space' to consciously monitor how you are feeling at each step of the routine. This is important, because you can get into the habit of defining each experience through emotions, words, and intuitive responses. These not only help you to better understand what you perceive, they will also develop your mastery of Celtic Reiki overall.

Once you are working regularly in the role of a Celtic Reiki professional, you will become increasingly comfortable with the idea of creating a more individual and personal connection to the Wise One, using your evolved responses as a guide.

THE WISE ONE CONNECTION TECHNIQUE:

1. Begin by sitting or standing in a comfortable position, ensuring your spine is upright, shoulders back, neck and head are aligned with your body and that you are facing straight ahead. Ensure your arms and legs are uncrossed, and if you are standing, have your feet a shoulder-width apart and your knees 'soft' (slightly bent, but still very supportive).

2. Focus on your breathing, by taking your attention to the effects of breath on the sides of your diaphragm, just below the ribcage and on your abdomen. The in-breath should cause you to expand out the sides and your tummy to rise. The out-breath contracts your sides and tummy, whilst you pull your lower abdominal muscles inwards (and when you are skilled, inwards and upwards). With each breath, count from the number one, upwards and trying to increase the count with each breath. Remember that the exhalation count should always be greater than the inhalation.

3. When you feel relaxed and internally-focused, state in your mind that this is to be a "connection to the Wise One Mystic" and then work through your Core State Visualisation.

4. In Core State, keep all images, 'screens', or thoughts that vie for your attention at a distance. Concentrate on simply being for a moment and then, locate the Wise One Mystic as a faraway star that glows brighter or a different colour from anything else.

5. Move the star towards you, keeping all else at bay

and paying attention to any other aspects of your surrounding environment that attempt to block you or limit you in any way. It is important to focus only on the 'star' as soon as you become aware of these other aspects.

6. Finally, connect to the star and step into your Wise One self. Experience the world in as much sensory depth as you can and ensure that you connect into their thought processes as often as possible. It may take a whilst to master the differentiation between the Wise One thoughts and other aspects of yourself, however this will become second-nature to you.

7. When you are ready to disconnect, simply thank the Wise One and visualise yourself stepping from the mystic and into your usual waking consciousness.

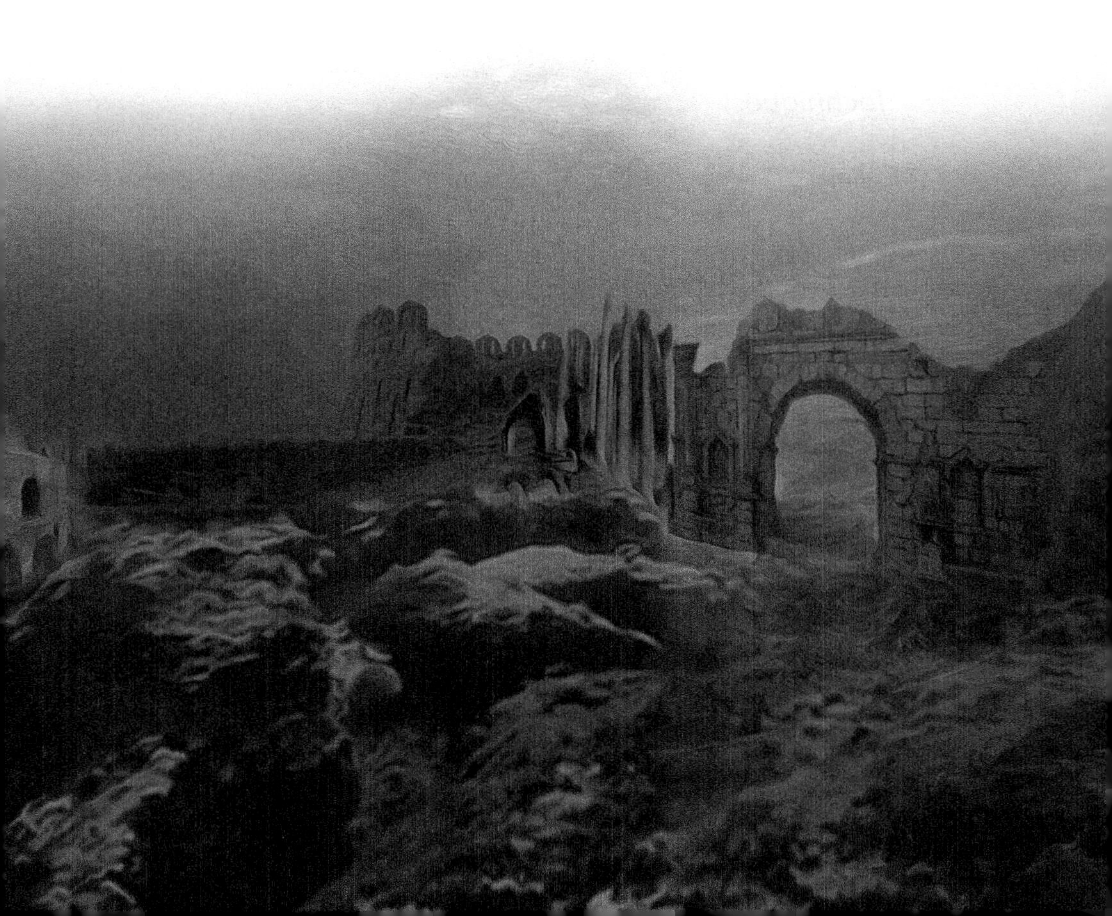

Realm Shifting with The Wise One

In the Adventurer's Guide, we examined how one can shift between realms with ease using the 'Realm Shifting' technique (p.113). Now we refine this process with particular emphasis on the qualities of the Wise One Mystic. This means that you will be able to shift between realms, whilst drawing-out the healing and compassionate thread that run through each realm.

For instance, the Furthest Ocean (which is associated with psychic and intuitive elements of Celtic Reiki) will be preserved at a base level, but also display a greater slant towards the interpretation of dis-ease and the psychic perception of client's issues during their treatment and consultation.

When Realm Shifting from the Wise One perspective, you will also concentrate the therapeutic features of essences from the Woodland, Standing Stones and Cosmic Realms. When shifting to the northern regions of the Mountain Range, the Master Mystic is usually favoured, however the Volcanic South will also display a greater degree of therapeutic shaping when shifted to, using the Wise One.

Technique:

1. Sitting or lying down with your arms and legs uncrossed and in a comfortable position, with your back straight, take your attention to your breathing. Take several deep breaths into your lower back and abdomen, using the same style of slow, regular breathing as you have done with the previous exercises.

2. With each exhalation, find yourself expanding and on every in-breath, 'fall' into yourself – not downwards, but inwards, as if flying to the centre or core of your being.

3. Internally, say that you are entering "Avatar State" and repeat the mantra "Wise One", three times, or use your favoured trigger method.

4. Feel the internal shifting from 'you', to 'you as the Mystic, Wise One'. Wait a few moments for this to occur then proceed.

5. Choose the first realm you want to work with—such as the Standing Stones, for instance—and internally, tell the Wise to "shift to the (x) realm" (where (x) is the chosen realm). As you do this, be aware of any changes in perception and note any synaesthesia responses you sense. I would recommend that you use your breath to 'slow' time whilst noticing the shift. This will enable you to squeeze the maximum amount of detail from the transition into the realm and you can then use this detail to recreate an instantaneous shift later.

6. Once you have entered the realm, use your senses to 'fine-tune' your experience of this particular realm. Does your inner vision become more colourful and sharp if you expand your awareness? If you shift your focus from left to right, do sounds become richer? How does it feel emotionally when you shape your internal position in relation to the realm? Use internal direction, position, focus, awareness, sense, etc. to monitor your synaesthesia and emotional responses and pay special attention to the experiences that seem 'better' in some way.

7. Once you have discovered your optimum realm experience, state internally to the Wise One Mystic that you want to go to the next realm (stating your second realm choice by name, for example, the Mountain Range).

8. As you shift, be absolutely aware of any sensations, synaesthetic reactions and notable experiences that you can use to recreate this transition at a later date. As you practise these shifts, your unconscious mind will monitor what you are doing and remember for future reference.

9. Once you have completed this for all five realms, come back into your conscious awareness of your physical environment and, when you are fully awake and focused, make notes on your experiences.

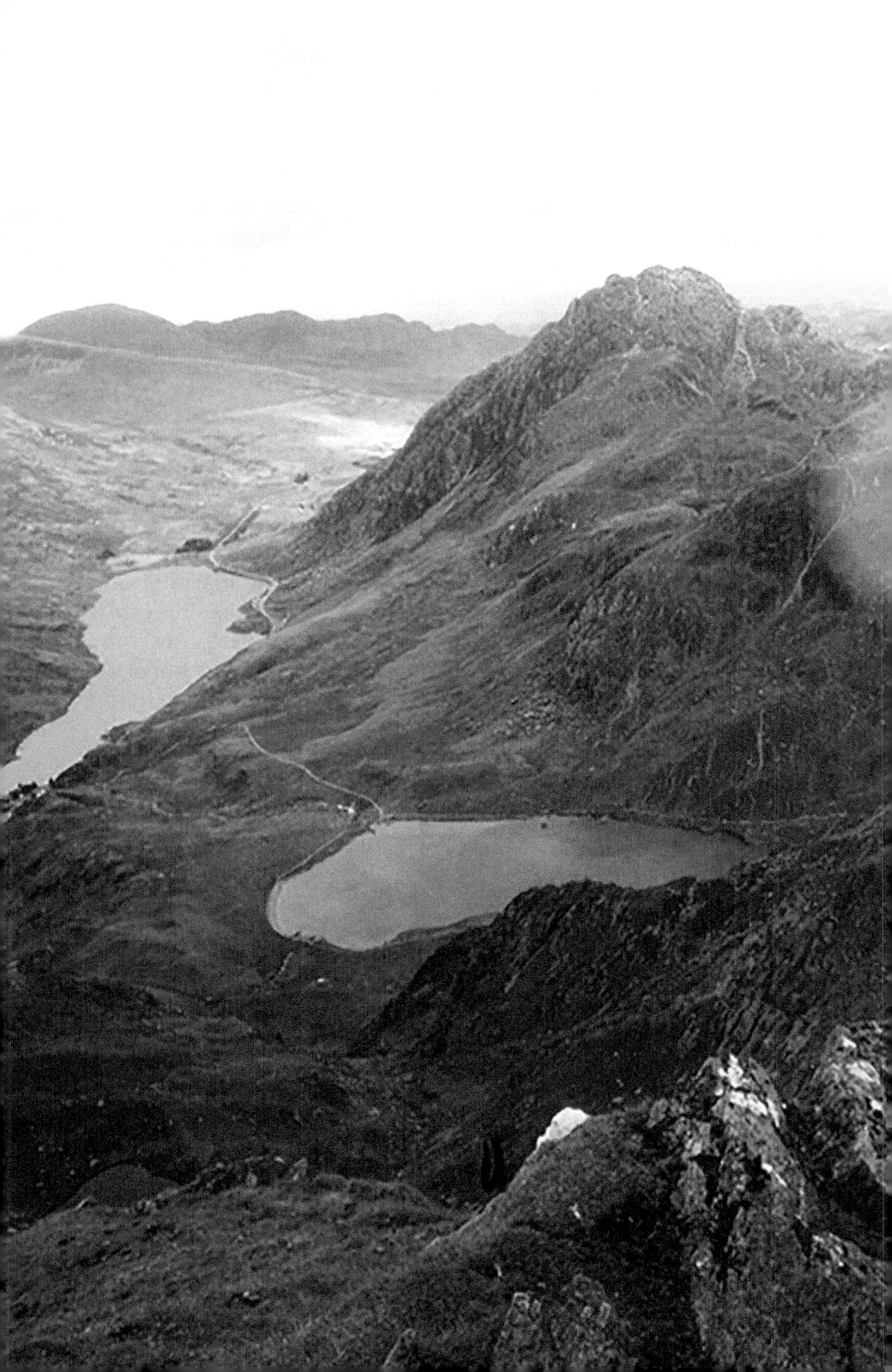

The Challenge of Wisdom

She watched as he came and stood near to her, drawn inexplicably to her like a moth that is captivated by moonlight. He appeared to be lost in thought, a trance that brought him closer to a source of light and healing, yet he remained completely unaware of his actions. She knew from her own path, how we are compelled to seek out what is most beneficial for us, yet often filter out that thing consciously. She had learnt to pay attention to these things: her subconscious actions; her body language; the phrases she used and statements she made. She would watch other people and hone in on groups, noticing the dynamics that formed as the individuals related to each other.

Without looking at the man, she shifted her perception to get as close to his as she could. The Wise One transitioned through waves of sensation, synaesthesia, emotion; all vaguely recognisable, yet distant. With each sensation, she focused her attention, brightening every colour, committing to every feeling. Each thought or seemingly random image had significance, so she dismissed nothing.

Collecting moments in this Technicolor, audio-kinaesthetic realm, she pieced together his story, his pain, his undoing...

How could a man feel so irredeemably lost? Alone in a world so full of people, stigmatised and outcast from a society full of those with lives just like him. Traumas and challenges, desires and joy, yet so removed by definition and label.

He has only ever wanted to be loved; to fall in love with another person and find a companion, with whom he could be himself. It was this search that had led him to find ways of numbing the pain. It was the numbness that drowned out the inner-voice... The only thing that has kept him going. It was not long before dis-ease came and the heartbreaking climb towards death became an inevitable path.

It was then he had met the love of his life - the prize that had evaded his life for so long. They had met in a local park on a sunny, mid-summer's day. Sitting, watching the trees and people going about their business; outsiders, observers, the watchers that sit beyond themselves and look with eyes that are greater than their own.

He had not noticed the man sitting on the bench adjacent to his own, until he had started to speak. He had been asking about the time and had seemed troubled, worried about some hidden challenge that time brought ever-closer. It was a simple question that heralded the thing he wanted for so long. In retrospect it seemed cruel that something so wished-for could be attained so easily, yet so long after hope had disappeared.

For many months they had met in the park, in the same place, at the same time of day, three, sometimes four times a week. It was in these moments they shared their lives, their passions, their achievements and their failures. It was here they fell in love.

For the first time in his life, the man had begun to believe in some greater force, a benevolence that had finally recognised his core need and had brought it to him. It was this overwhelming sense of being embraced by an intelligent force, beyond himself that gave him the courage to hope once again. Maybe he could find forgiveness for all he had done? Perhaps this life of darkness and hurt was not meant to be his legacy? Could it be that the dis-ease that was turning his own body against itself, wasting him away in nothingness, slowly sapping the very essence of his will to go on, would not be his only companion? For if he died, knowing he was loved by another, that would not be a death at all... It would be a release from the walking death he had been living for so long.

It was with this euphoria, this joyful, fleeting, and fragile moment of time that he simply burst with happiness. He felt that constant weight that had beared down upon him for so many years, lift and for the first time in his lonely life, he had a companion that was so much more than drugs and pain and death. It was not long after that, that the his companion stopped coming to their meetings and the man realised he would never see him again.

As she unravelled his story, she felt a pang of sadness. For she walked a fine line between what is and what she defined the world to be. The Wise One knew that this terrible loss, this trauma must exist within her own perception of the world, for her to acknowledge it in another. Now that she had connected into this part of herself, she had defined another person in such a way as this. She knew that she must find a way of healing the situation: for herself and that hidden aspect of her being, who felt so unlovable, so utterly forsaken; and for the man who had come into her life and offered her the opportunity to heal through his suffering.

As the man moved off, down the aisle, she took a deep breath and deliberated on how best to begin...

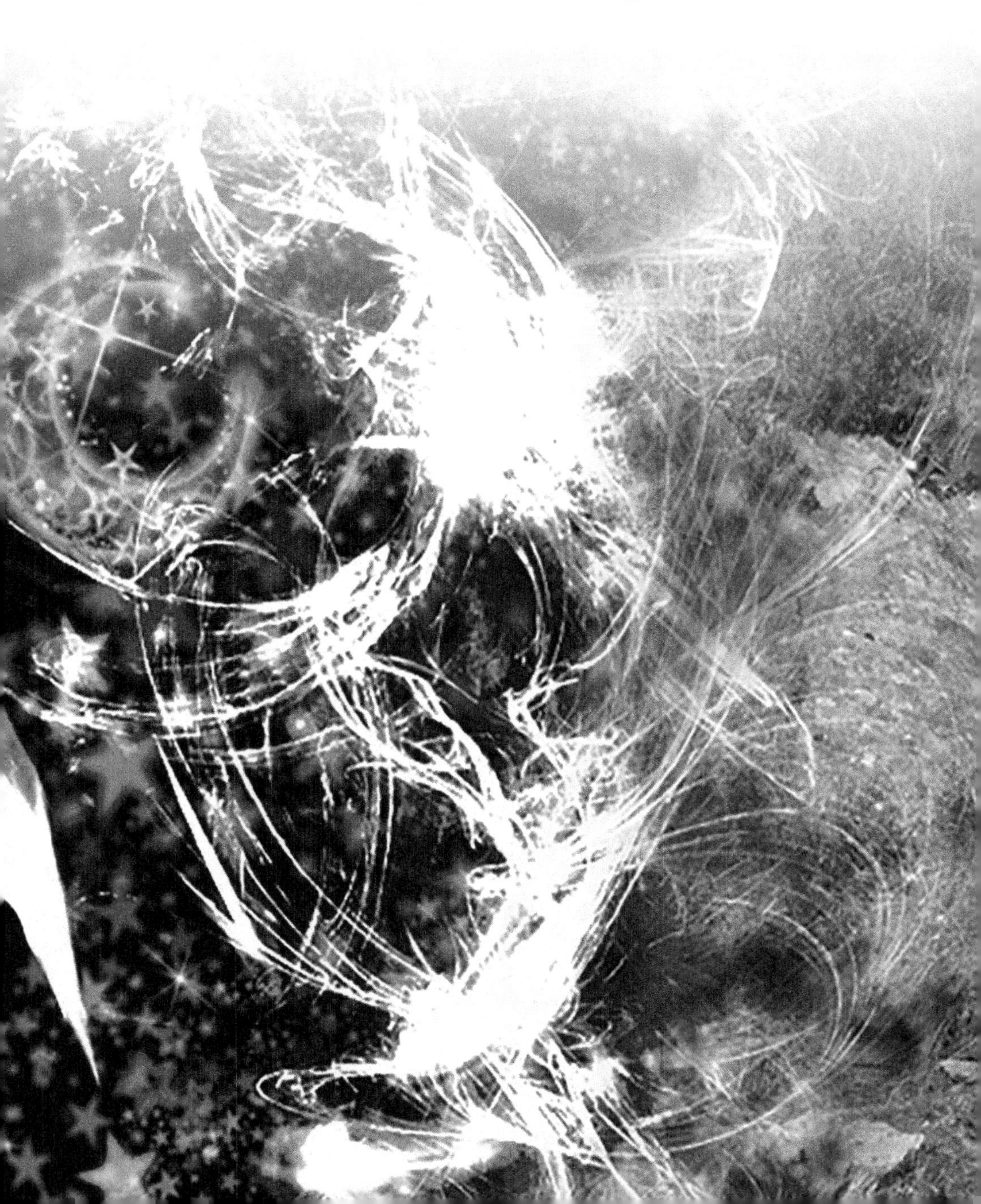

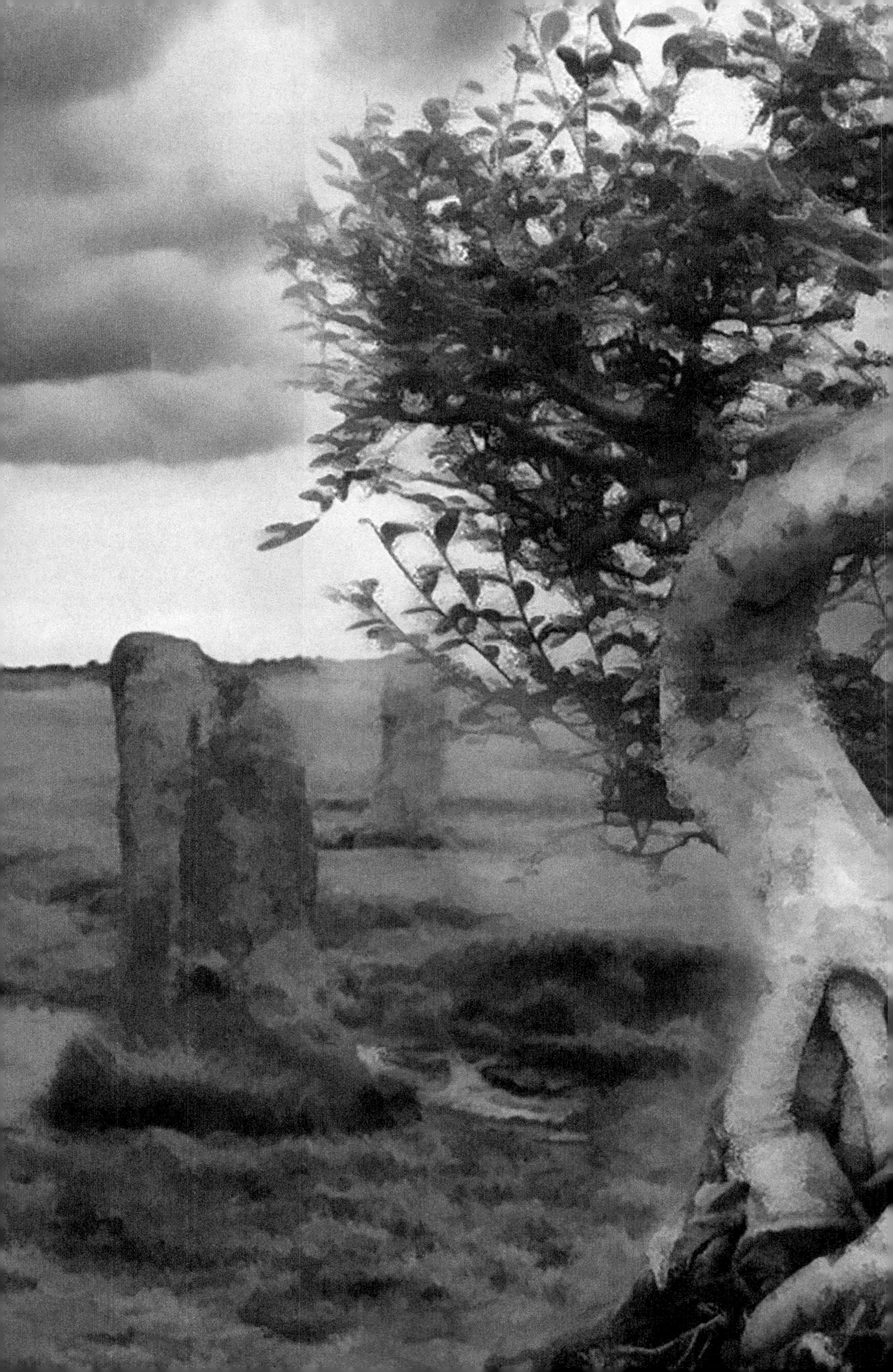

Treatment Methods of the Wise One

Selestrhy and Fwddiau

The Wise One views these two methods as the cornerstones of Celtic Reiki from a therapeutic perspective. Selestrhy (Sell-less-tr-hee) and Fwddiau (Vowed-thee-eye) mean, respectively: the Heavens and the Void. The Wise One uses both as 'scanning' and treatment styles that focus on the intuitive application of Celtic Reiki (Selestrhy) and the enhancement of sensitivity to vibrational change (Fwddiau).

In other words, use of Selestrhy creates intuitive or psychic awareness and Fwddiau will help you to distinguish different essences, vibrational issues, etc. As you slip into Avatar State and work as the Wise One, you develop your skills. These techniques can lead to some amazing sensory abilities, such as, knowledge of future events in relation to your clients and the effect of perceiving your client's diseases, just by looking at them.

These easy to use, yet incredibly powerful techniques are so varied in results and potent in effect that you could actually build your entire practice style, based solely on these alone. Both offer the possibility for detailed feedback from your client and your own synaesthetic responses.

Selestrhy and Fwddiau have many uses, which include: intuitive knowledge of a client's physical health; improving emotional and cerebral wellbeing; clearing ancestral trauma; and even improving prophetic ability with relation to your client's future. Yet they are both empowered through combination with essences and shaping skills. Here, Selestrhy and Fwddiau come into their own; helping the Practitioner to master the different essences in preparation for teaching and harvesting.

SELESTRHY—THE HEAVENS

Beginning with Selestrhy, which embodies the shifting of the Heavens, the fluidity of the air and all the potential of the Universe, the hands (and eventually the mental focus) of the Practitioner are used to sense the dynamic patterns of the client's bioenergetic field. Resembling a graceful dance, the Celtic Reiki Practitioner is guided to work at various points, where gentle stroking, energetic swirling, dynamic pulsing and balletic finger movements take place.

Without volition or conscious intervention, the Practitioner can concentrate on the myriad joys of internal sensation and imagery as they relax and let their intuitive, subconscious perform a powerful treatment. Often accompanied with a brilliant 'light show' of shapes and coloured light, this remarkable technique is one of the simplest to conduct.

Technique:

1. To conduct a Selestrhy treatment, simply start with a connection to your client by placing your hands either side of their head, about an inch or two away from their temples (without touching their head). There will be an internal shift of sensation, after which, state in your mind that you are going to treat your subject with Selestrhy.

2. When you feel a good connection to Celtic Reiki (with or without triggering named essences), move to the side of your subject and place your hands over their abdominal region. Continue to nurture your connection to Reiki until your hands begin to move to a new position; this will feel like a magnetic pull or push and can be disconcerting at first, but just allow this to happen. It is important not to make a change happen, or resist the movement when it does – just go with the flow!

3. If your hands move to their fullest extent, feel free to travel around your subject to obtain a more comfortable position for yourself. Remain at each position until your hands once again move of their own accord.

4. At the end of the treatment, go to your subject's head area and finish with a final head connection.

Fwddiau—The Void

Fwddiau is the Void, although rather than a complete non-existence of anything, the Void in Celtic Reiki is a lack of vibrational potency or some form of distortion. These form a void in certain areas of the wellbeing of a client. Healing the Void, through scanning, sensing and treatment (of affected dynamics) promotes health for your client and a heightened degree of sensitivity in your energy-awareness abilities.

The Void effects that are sensed by Fwddiau are a wide range of sensations that will affect your hands, arms and other parts of your body, internally and even 'around' your body. These effects can be heat, icy cold, itching, formication (the sensation of insects crawling across the skin), spasms/twitching muscles, stabbing, tickling, breezes, and many other unusual feelings. Each of these represents a different type of distortion in your client's bioenergetic field and can be related to some physical or emotional dis-ease.

As you scan for Void effects, you will discover how to recognise these through sight, sound, taste and smell, as well as at a direct, vibrational level. Upon clearing the effects, you heal the associated dis-ease they are connected to.

Technique:

1. To conduct a treatment using Fwddiau, simply start by connecting to Celtic Reiki via a 'head connection': place your hands either side of your subject's head and feel an internal shifting, as with Selestrhy.

2. Then use your non-dominant hand to 'scan' your subject's body, sensing the Void sensations in the aura/bioenergetic field surrounding the body. Upon discovering a Void effect, focus Celtic Reiki essences of your choosing at the location until the Void has ceased or 10 minutes have passed.

3. Upon clearing the Void, repeat the scanning until you

have located and cleared as many effects as possible in the treatment time.

4. Complete the treatment with a final head connection and then bring your subject back into the room.

Harmonics and Pure Essences

The concept of the harmonic had been adapted over the years to evolve into a finely nuanced philosophy. The initial idea was that an essence would contain harmonics or 'noise', which could be used 'as is' or stripped away to create a 'pure essence'. An example of this would be an essence harvested from a single Rowan tree - the pure essence would be Luis, however, without any form of stripping, the essence would contain much of the individual tree's perspective.

The core ideals of harmonics still remain in Celtic Reiki, with greater emphasis on 'viewpoint' than originally presented. Since its inception, the inclusion of additional perspectives have created a much wider scope for the stripping processes, for we now take into consideration the harvester and other factors, such as location, etc.

Ultimately, these other factors have a bearing on the individuals of each essence, which can be stripped from the essence to form an essence of the foundation species, type, class, etc. What has shifted our view considerably is that all essences will be affected by the harvester (except in the case of those harvested using Viridian Methodology). This translates to every essence being from the perspective of the person who harvested it, as opposed to some 'pure' or 'Universal' essence.

Therefore, the closest you can have to a 'pure essence' is one that you have harvested yourself and that has been stripped to its most basic form. The results of stripping tend to be essences that have a greater degree of effect on ever-increasing layers of perception.

So, a good rule of thumb would be that an essence without any stripping tends to work more physically - has the greatest physical action and lasts for the shortest period (hours or days). The first stripping will take an essence to a more emotional place and create a longer lasting period of activity (days to weeks), whilst a further stripping lasts longer (weeks to a month) and focuses on cerebral challenges. A final stripping will have an immense effect, spiritually and last for several months —though it will tend to offer little conscious sensation or result.

This leads to very few noticeable sensations or experiences with an essence that is fully stripped of harmonics and often means that practitioners avoid any more than two stripping sessions. However, if you are confident in your treatment methods, and have a client with whom you have a good rapport, you can fully strip an essence for remarkably deep-acting and long-lasting results.

STRIPPING THE HARMONICS

The process of stripping the harmonics of an essence is very simple and can be conducted during the treatment or practice, immediately before 'application'. How many times you strip the essence will depend on the goals you wish to achieve, however, once or twice is the preferred amount, with three strips being reserved for the most deep-acting of treatments.

Technique:

1. Connect to the essence you require and feel it in your head, your hands and your arms.
2. Close your eyes and visualise a wall of light emanating from you.
3. Imagine this light getting 'thinner' in width – not lessening the strength of the sensation, but reducing the actual 'thickness' of the wall.
4. When you feel this reach a single line, you have reached the emotional level.
5. Expand the light again, keeping the sensation created by the vibration the same.
6. Repeat [3 & 4] to reach the cerebral level.
7. To go to a spiritual level, you can repeat [3 & 4] one more time to reach the pure essence and this will work very deeply on you and your client, altering deeply rooted trauma, etc.

An Essence for Each Season

Many practitioners regard essences as mirroring the cycles of the seasons and the Celtic calendar. This idea is very much down to 'taste' and will depend on your personal viewpoint as to its effectiveness. However in simple terms – the Evergreen trees are more potent in winter, the Deciduous trees in summer and the emphasis changes in each essence throughout the year – the cycle of Ruis, for example, is more relevant to 'preparation for change' in spring, and the 'accepting of change' in autumn.

You will also find that at some times, particular essences are stronger overall than at other times of year – this is because their resonance is in accordance with your resonance. Make notes of these shifts in a diary and you will soon see a pattern emerge. Use this to find your preferred essences for use at their most potent times of year. There should be one, possibly several essences per month – use these (at peak times) as much as possible on yourself and on others for even better results.

Some Masters believe the season is irrelevant to the potency of an essence, because it is winter (or summer, spring, autumn) somewhere on the Earth throughout the year. It is always winter from an Earth-wide perspective, however, this is an intellectual perspective, not experiential. As essences are so reliant on the perspectives of practitioner, master, and client, this needs to be taken into consideration when working at different times.

Make notes about your particular sensations with particular essences at different times of year, as this will display what is the best approach for you as an individual.

A Forest of perspective

The Treatment Forest is a simple to use and very effective way of combining perspectives into one, smooth and congruent essence. When treating with several essences, a treatment can become 'bitty' and lose its focus, as the addition of each new perspective creates a 'meandering' through the forest that results in losing one's way! The Treatment Forest, however, harmonises the various essences, orientating them in the direction of the desired results.

This translates to the scenario of being the forest, rather than merely finding one's way through it. An active approach to treatment that places Practitioner and client in a more assertive positive. There is a tendency to view essences as being 'outside' of oneself and 'bigger' than oneself - yet every person has many perspectives of their own.

The art of the Treatment Forest simply translates a person's own perspectives to those of the particular forest. Comparing the perspective of treatment to our personal perspectives does not diminish the power of the treatment - it reminds each of us of how we constantly belittle the power of the self and just how much we are personally capable of.

An example of a Treatment Forest, is BRANCH (Beith, Ruis, Ailim, Coll, Huathe). This would be the perspective of beginnings, because the forest essence is Birch. Hence there is a suggestion of initiation here, new projects or the next chapter in a person's life.

It could also be a treatment for a client who is pregnant or wants to conceive. As with all essences, remember to glean your own understanding of each essence, because everybody has their own view of individual essences that alters results from person to person.

Next comes Ruis, which highlights legal matters, amongst other things, maybe this treatment is to help set up a business and dealing with the legalities of the process. It could also be used to resolve custody issues if used in pregnancy or perhaps help a mother who is fighting for her rights and those of her child. Ailim adds foresight and vision to the treatment; instilling a sense of business acumen to the entrepreneur or offering a mother-to-be a sense of knowing, understanding, and 'home'.

This process works for the entire forest and is usually constructed from feedback given by the client. As they express their dis-eases, challenges, and desired results for the treatment, the Wise One will apportion an essence to each aspect of the treatment. They then examine their list of essences for those which appear more than once - Nuin is the 'Keeper of Secrets' and also helps to heal hidden dis-ease (without diagnosis or obvious 'root cause').

One they have decided upon essences - through relevance to the client's needs, frequency of occurrence (how many times it appears in the Wise One's prescription), and intuition - the Wise One will decide upon a handful (between four and six essences) for use as the forest.

The Treatment Forest is very easy to create and makes an excellent companion for a Selestrhy treatment. Simply state at the begining of treatment that this is to be a 'Treatment Forest' and then trigger each essence in turn, using your preferred method of trigger (Ogham, visual symbol, mantra, intent, etc.). Then continue with the treatment as usual, using hand positions, Selestrhy, or other treatment technique of your choosing. Finally, complete the treatment, thanking each essence and whomever else you wish to offer gratitude to.

Treatment Forest can be used for any Tree Essence, remembering that Non-Celtic Trees have no letter associations and therefore, do not create 'words'. With this in mind, you may also choose to adapt the Treatment Forest for use with essences outside the Woodland Realm, although in these instances, you may prefer another technique that is well suited to the layering of perspective - The Woodhenge.The Treatment Forest & The Woodhenge

All treatments, routines, and methods in Celtic Reiki are derived by definition. The style in which a practice is defined will form the basis for its effectiveness and the results achieved. The more clarity you can instil within the parameters of a treatment, the greater the results.

Whenever you conduct a treatment, you are often wise to limit the number of vibrations you use at any one time, as using many different essences can cause your definition to become fragmented. This will make a treatment seem 'bitty' and without a solid, definitive focus. To avoid this happening, the Treatment Forest can be used to plant essences into a clearly defined 'set' of intents and create a forest (Stone Circle, etc.) that can be used as a single essence, thus replacing many.

The concept of a Treatment Forest is very useful, especially when treating people who require many different essences to assist in easing their various situations and diseases. Yet the forest is always different, because each, individual tree lends itself to a whole, thus an autonomous forest has many unique dynamics and qualities. Next time you walk through a wood, try to sense the energy of the woodland as a whole and then communicate with the individual trees and see the difference – although each tree is part of the whole, the forest is a complete contrast; greater than a combination of single trees.

Consequently, how do you use many different essences in a treatment, keeping a strong intent and focus, yet maintaining the integrity of each individual tree essence? For the answer to this, we look to another form of therapy and the personal development system known as The Viridian Method. In the methodology of VM is a technique known as Parallel Projection, which is translated for Celtic Reiki practice to the Woodhenge (or Stonehenge, if working within the Standing Stones Realm).

The Woodhenge is the technique by which Woodland Realm essences can be stacked into a single treatment essence, yet maintain all of the original qualities. This works on the basis that each single essence is defined in the same place, at the same time, yet in different layers of perception.

To grasp this, imagine that you walk through a forest, taking a path that leads you past many different trees. At various points along the path you stop and interact with an individual tree.

Now in your linear perspective, you experience this journey as 'one tree after another', however if you step outside of time, all the interactions occur without a time distinction. In other words, it is like reading a book—all the events exist in the book, though the linear journey of reading the book is necessary for you to become consciously aware of those events!

The creation of the Woodhenge is where you simply define a set of parameters with a specific structure. In energetic terms, you split your client throughout several realities, treat them with a single essence in each reality and them 'put them back together' in this reality.

Without getting too technical, this process is based

upon a parallel with the principle of 'Photon Duality'; a concept in Quantum philosophy.

This is where a particle of light (Photon) can exist in two different places at the same time if it possible for it to do so. If you create more possible paths for the photon to travel along, it will do this also—all at the same time! It truly is possible for the photon to be in two places at once!

Of course the process is much simpler in practice than it may sound here, because you only need define a treatment as "The Woodhenge" and then activate each essence you wish to add to the treatment.

Once you have done this, simply continue with the treatment style you have chosen as you would normally. The thing to remember is that you can place several (all, if you wish) treatment essences into a single Woodhenge and treat your subject for a whole hour—every time you add an essence, they will be technically receiving their hour treatment, multiplied by the number of essences!

So if you use five essences in a Woodhenge treatment, you are offering your client five hours of treatment in just one hour of time!

The Stargate Trinity Treatment

Continuing the theme of 'henges', this treatment method uses the Stargate (Stonehenge) Essence to form a gateway between the Earth and some cosmic destination. Here you choose the crystal type, from which you would like to construct your Stonehenge/Stargate and a destination essence (usually a Stellar or Planetary Essence).

Technique:

1. Lay your client on the treatment couch, or sit them in a padded chair, ensuring that they are comfortable. If you are conducting a self-treatment, simply sit in a chair or lie down with your open palms on your body.
2. Close your eyes and make a head connection by placing your hands either side of your client's temples – near the skin, but without touching.

3. Activate the first essence, which will be a Crystal Essence of your choosing. Your hands can remain at the same position throughout the treatment, or you can move them as you intuit.

4. Maintain this connection for 3-5 minutes before triggering the Stargate Essence and continue to hold this perspective for a further 3-5 minutes.

5. Now activate the third and final trigger, which will be your chosen Stellar Essence. At this point you may wish to guide your client through a meditation, or, if self-treating, use visual imagery to heighten your experience. Continue at the level of these three essences for the duration of the treatment.

6. Once you have conducted the treatment for the desired time, bring your client back into the room and offer them some water to drink.

7. Ensure they are fully aware and comfortable before asking them to stand up.

Shaping Essences

As soon as you have Calibrated to the Wise One Orientation, you will be able to work well with the following techniques. Indeed, the shaping routines can be used after even the basic Orientations or 'attainments', yet the Wise One Mystic is particularly masterful when creatively shaping a perspective to specific needs.

If you are experiencing these exercises whilst working with the Adventurer Mystic, or you are approaching them for the first time, as the Wise One, you can maximise your success by ensuring that you complete each one in turn and then only move on after you feel completely comfortable.

These shaping methods are also available in essence form, therefore offering you the choice of defining the shapes anew for each client, or of using a set of pre-constructed definitions that present the perspective of each shape (The Encyclopaedia of Celtic Reiki Essences, mPowr.)

Exercise One—Line or Spiral

In this simple exercise, stand in front of a person or object and visualise yourself directing an essence at them. You can use your hands if it focuses your intent, or just 'beam' it at the object.

Once you have done this, attempt to beam energy in a straight line at an imaginary object, or distant place/event.

If you wish, you can try 'spiralling' the energy outwards from you at the centre to the outermost point of the spiral, the object (this intensifies the resulting dynamic). An interesting version of this is to imagine energy spiralling in at you and see the effect!

Exercise Two—Triangle

This exercise works with a challenge or issue that you have in your life currently. Stand in an open space and imagine the problem diagonally to your right. Imagine that you are beaming Reiki or light at it, as you did with Exercise One.

See energy burst through the problem and turn to the left, where it starts to create a solution. Then bring this solution to you, diagonally from the left hand side.

Exercise Three—Square

For this exercise, you can use a desired goal that is either blocked by two conflicting issues (challenges), or two imagined objects (such as pillars or even people).

The goal could be, for example, that you want to write a book, although your job does not allow you the time—if you leave your job, you will not have enough money to support yourself.

Visualise the two challenges, or objects on each diagonal to you, and then imagine you are directing Reiki/light at them simultaneously.

Watch energy work through the two points and then converge on a point opposite you to form a square.

If you wish, you can then imagine yourself at the opposite point, soaking up the energy of your goal.

Exercise Four – Cube

This exercise is a little more complex and involves multiple 'targets', so for ease of learning, you can imagine three people; two diagonally from you, and one diagonally from them – opposite you.

You want to 'beam' Reiki at the person in front of you, but cannot, so imagine two streams of energy coming from your feet and beam these either side of you, to the 'diagonal people'. Then produce similar streams at head level and see all four beams working through the two people. The energy intensifies and is then directed at the focus person opposite you.

With practice, you will be able to substitute the two diagonally positioned people for up to 4 conflicting issues and then see a single solution opposite.

When you feel that the Reiki or light has reached the solution, see yourself standing in the opposite position 'soaking up the energy'. If you are finding that the problems are overwhelming you, you can then visualise yourself in the centre of the cube, unaffected by the challenges.

Intuition of the Wise One

Technique:

1. Stand in the centre of a room in a quiet place where you will not be disturbed for the duration of the exercise.

2. Centre yourself, close your eyes and bring your focus inwards.

3. Turn your attention completely to your breathing, taking long, slow, deep breaths that cause your stomach to expand and chest to move outwards to the sides.

4. Breathe this way until you start to feel relaxed and very calm – if you feel dizzy or light-headed, sit down for a while until you feel better.

5. Place your hands out in front of you, palms facing

down and start to project a Celtic Reiki essence, such as Saille or Duir, while pushing downwards through the air.

6. When you reach a resistance, 'sit' your hands on this 'energy cushion' and relax your arms into this resting place. If you wish, you can ask in your mind for your guides to be with you or ask for assistance from your 'higher-self'. Many people do find additional help very useful at this point and who you ask for help is entirely up to you. You may want to ask for unseen friends, your loved ones who have passed over, nature spirits or other spiritual beings. You might also decide that you prefer just to work on your own, in which case, ask to connect to your 'higher levels of consciousness'.

7. Now affirm that you will experience 'the vibrations of this location through my subtle senses' and wait for a response. This response should take the form of a slight 'magnetic' pull in your hands, which should direct one or both of your hands to the left/right. You may also find this sensation pulling you forward or backward and do be prepared for this with 'soft knees'. If the pull takes you beyond the comfortable reach of your arms, you can walk slowly in the desired direction. It is important to use the word 'location' rather than saying 'the room' as you are sensing our energetic place as opposed to the physical locale.

8. Search for changes in the vibrations and continue to explore these changes until you find a vibration so 'heavy' that you cannot push through it without using muscle effort.

9. Bounce your hands along these heavy vibrations until you have a good idea of the boundaries.

10. Push your hands further into the vibrations of energy —if the force is too strong and pushes you back, or resists completely, push the fingertips of your left hand into the barrier, creating a claw with your hand that pierces the energy instead of pushing.

11. Ask in your mind, what 'this' is and then clear your mind as best you can.

12. Allow images, words, feelings, sounds and so on, to fill your mind. You might find it helps at this point to clarify what you perceive by stating aloud your experiences.

13. Upon completing this, come fully back into the room, take a seat and have a moment to compose yourself and make any notes.

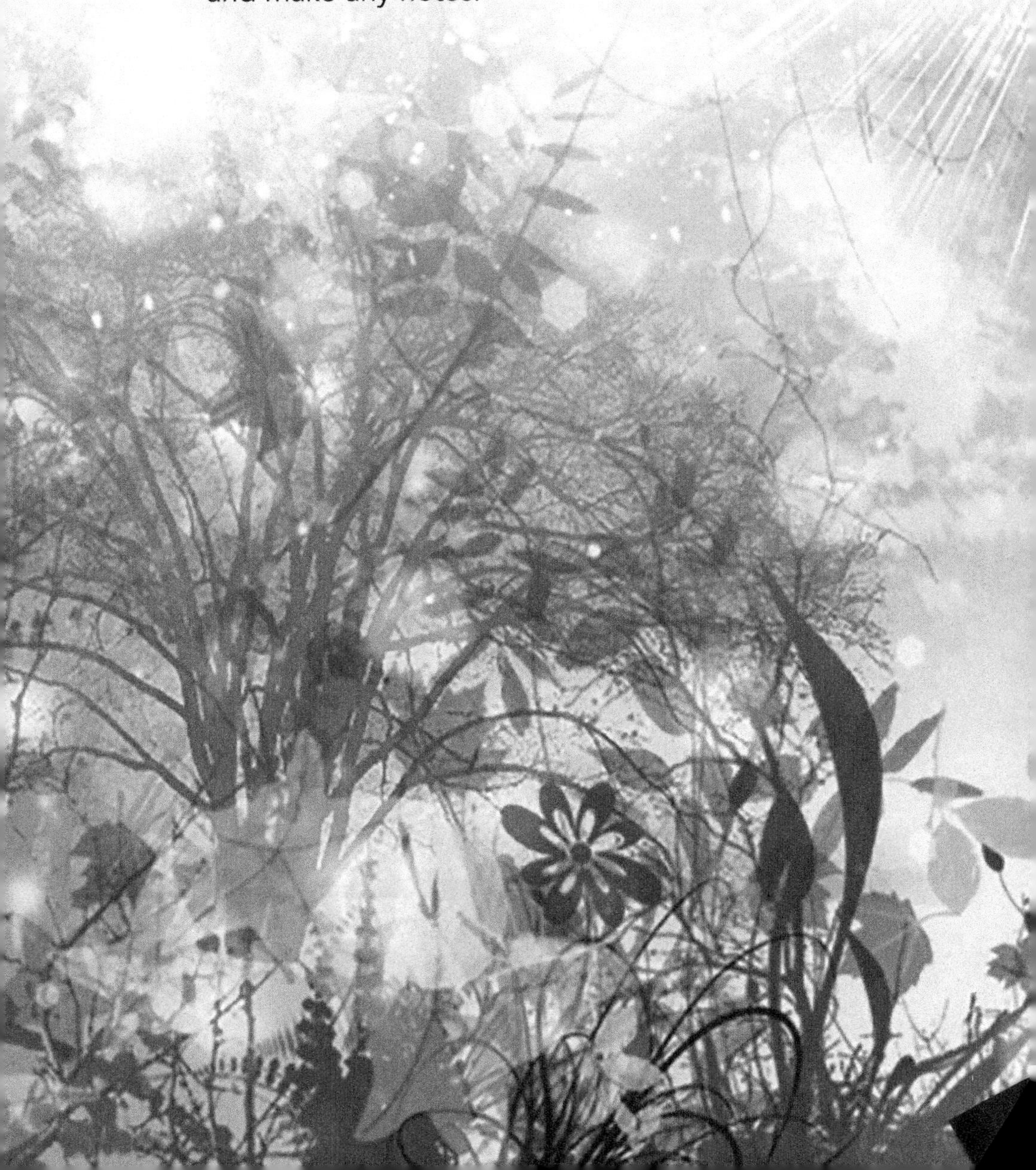

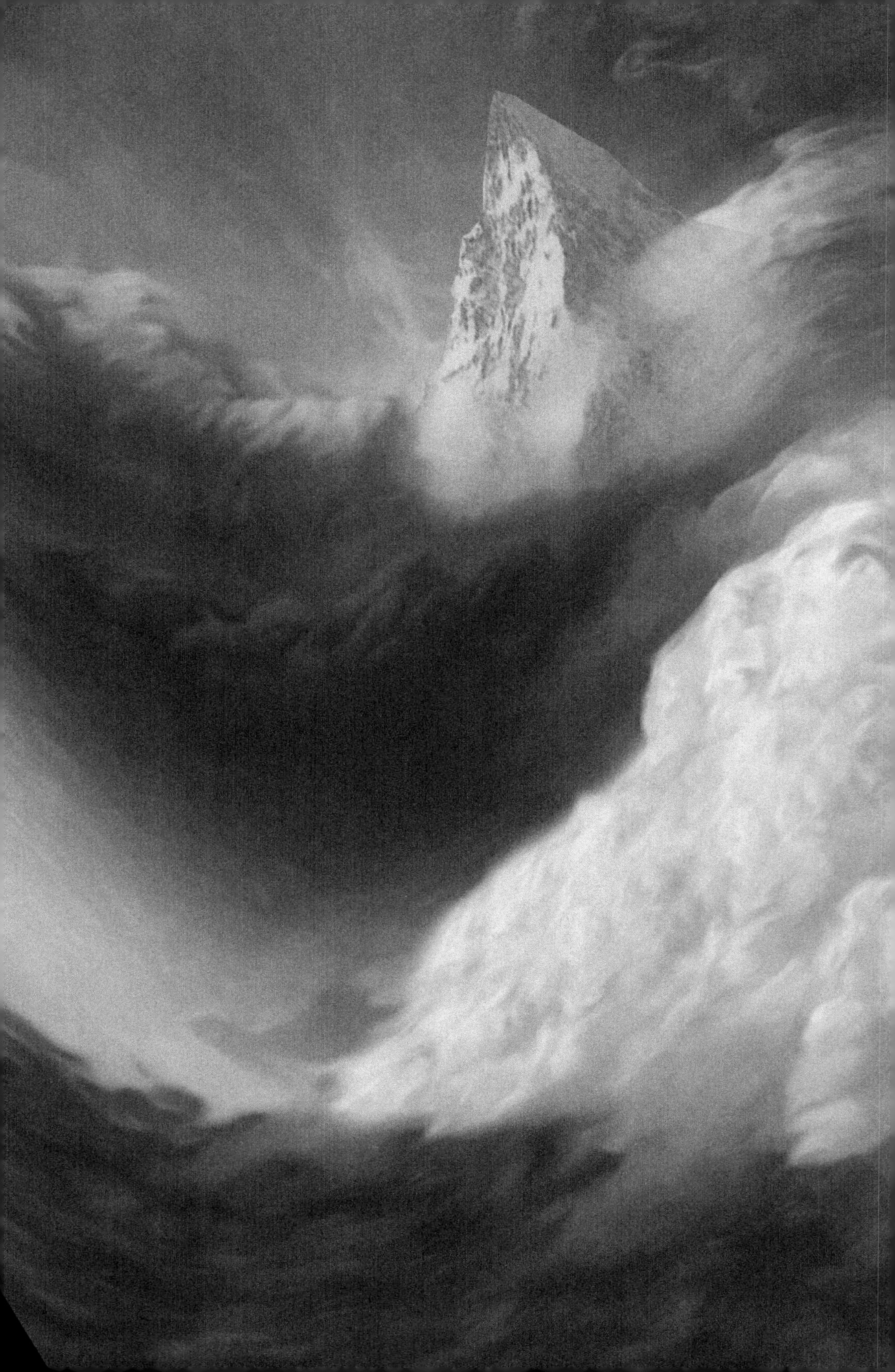

RAISING THE FIRE

This form of treatment is an excellent motivator and invigorator, as it stimulates energy to very high levels thus raising the effectiveness of a treatment with people who tend towards the lowering of vibrations, for example, those who suffer with depression, ME, lethargy, etc. This treatment is particularly expansive for clients who feel great for around two hours after treatment, but then return to the previous state.

A vital aspect to remember with Fire is that, in Eastern philosophy, Fire and Wood are linked, Wood feeds Fire, yet Fire destroys Wood. I have often found this in the treatment as we start with your chosen tree essences that slowly subside to the Tan Essence. Do not worry about the trees, as this does not affect them at all – it is a purely energetic effect of the treatment!

By instilling tree essences at the beginning of the treatment, you will have an effect on your client that is identical to a normal Celtic Reiki treatment using those essences. However, once you raise the fire, the tree elements will give way to a very powerful stimulation of energy (Fire) that will create vigour and dynamic potential in the tree essences. By the completion of the treatment, your client will feel invigorated, yet the tree essences will still be underlying and working away to achieve the intent of the treatment.

Therefore, rather than a common scenario in these circumstances where the tree essences work for a while before easing back to the previous state, here the fire will keep your client's energy levels high so that the tree essences can work for longer and more efficiently.

Technique:

1. Start using your breath and favoured visualisation to shift into Core State and then connect to the Wise One Mystic.
2. Now, state internally, this is to be a "Raising the Fire

Treatment".

3. Stand at your client's head, with your hands at their temples and activate your chosen Woodland Realm essences either as a Treatment Forest or in a Woodhenge.

4. Once you have a good sense of the essences, just relax and let the energy build. Remain for 10 minutes at the head area and then for a further 10 minutes on the shoulders.

5. Now move to the side of your client and complete a further 10 minutes with one hand over your subject's heart and the other at the base (pelvic) area.

6. 30 minutes into the treatment, you begin to Raise the Fire with the activation of Tan.

7. Imagine your hands are resting on a carpet of energy, just above your client, in a position, where you are resting your arms comfortably on this carpet instead of holding them there. Relax your shoulders.

8. Now allow your arms and hands to move along the perceived waves of magnetism, going to whatever area of your subject's body or aura they wish to move to. Whilst doing this, imagine flames of energy glowing with the colours of the rainbow, flickering up from your client's body to meet your hands. Feel the heat of these flames against the palms of your hands.

9. Continue this for a further 20-30 minutes, seeing the flames becoming more and more vibrant as they completely encompass your subject and glow brighter and brighter.

10. At the end of the treatment, make a final 'head connection' with your client (hands on the temples), thank the Wise One and then work through any usual closing routine that you have.

11. Bring your subject into the room, make sure they are lucid and then offer them some water to drink!

THE BREATH OF WIND

This technique uses the element of Air to create an energy dynamic that is gentle, yet multifaceted in effect, and all-encompassing. The routine is very relaxing, for both the client and the practitioner, as you gently stimulate your client's energetic systems with Celtic Reiki essences, your breath, and slow, repetitive movements. Particularly good for people with lots of stress and tension, the Breath of Wind helps people to lift upwards and focus forwards, rather than focusing themselves into the ground.

This is an excellent method for people who are 'too grounded' and look only to the physical for every solution and when making decisions. I have also found this form of treatment works well on the symptoms of dis-eases created as a result of this attitude.

These can be, but are not limited to, cancer, neurological illness, hypertension and the effects caused by heart-attack or stroke. The technique is also wonderful for people who are 'stuck' emotionally, or in states where they lack emotion or experience emotional stagnation – such as people stuck in relationships or life situations that are no longer serving them in beneficial ways.

The Wind rustles the branches and leaves of the trees, enabling them to sing to each other and communicate using murmured messages that are carried on the breeze.

Hence, this method can also be valuable when wanting to stimulate the creativity of energy, causing it to 'sing' with vibrancy or to work with affirmations for your subject that can be formed through the initial consultation, or through the use of affirmation cards.

Technique

1. Take several long, deep breaths and then shifting yourself into Core State. When completely at one, in your Core State, connect to the Wise One Mystic.

2. In your mind, state that this is to be a "Breath of Wind Treatment".

3. Stand at your subject's head, with your hands at their temples and activate your chosen essences as a

Treatment Forest or in the Woodhenge.

4. Once you have a good sense of energy, just relax and let the energy build, holding conscious attention on the rhythm of your breathing. Take long slow breaths, whilst visualising yourself pulling in the energy of Annal and exhaling this energy on your breath. This should be blown out through your mouth so slowly and gently that your subject cannot feel it, yet it acts like the wind in their energy field.

5. Continue this for 10 minutes, easing your breath if you become faint or dizzy. Then continue at the shoulders for a further 10 minutes.

6. Now, remaining at your subject's head area, lift your hands so that they are about 12 inches above their head, palms facing downwards. Then slowly sweep the air down the length of their body so that your arms stretch forward completely and your palms are facing away from you – breathe out as you do this. Breathe in and return your palms to their original position. Repeat for 10 minutes.

7. Then go to the side of your subject and stand at the midpoint of their body, around the lower abdomen. Place your hands, palms down, at their head area and then breathing out as you do so, sweep your hands slowly, steadily and gently down the length of your subject's body until you reach their feet (or as close as you can get to their feet without moving). Breathe in as you return your hands to the head area and pull in Annal as you do so.

8. After 10 minutes, go down to your client's feet and repeat the exercise listed in (6) the head area section, except this time, come up the body with your sweeping hands. Do this for 10 minutes.

9. Now go to the other side of your client and stand at their midpoint. Place your hands palms facing down at your subject's feet (or as best you can without overreaching) and slowly sweep energy up their body

to their head (or as near as you can). Breathe out as you do this and breathe in as you return your hands to the feet.

10. At the end of the treatment, make a final head connection with your subject (hands on the temples), silently express your gratitude to the Wise One and then work through your usual closing routine.

11. Bring your subject into the room, make sure they are lucid, and then offer them some water.

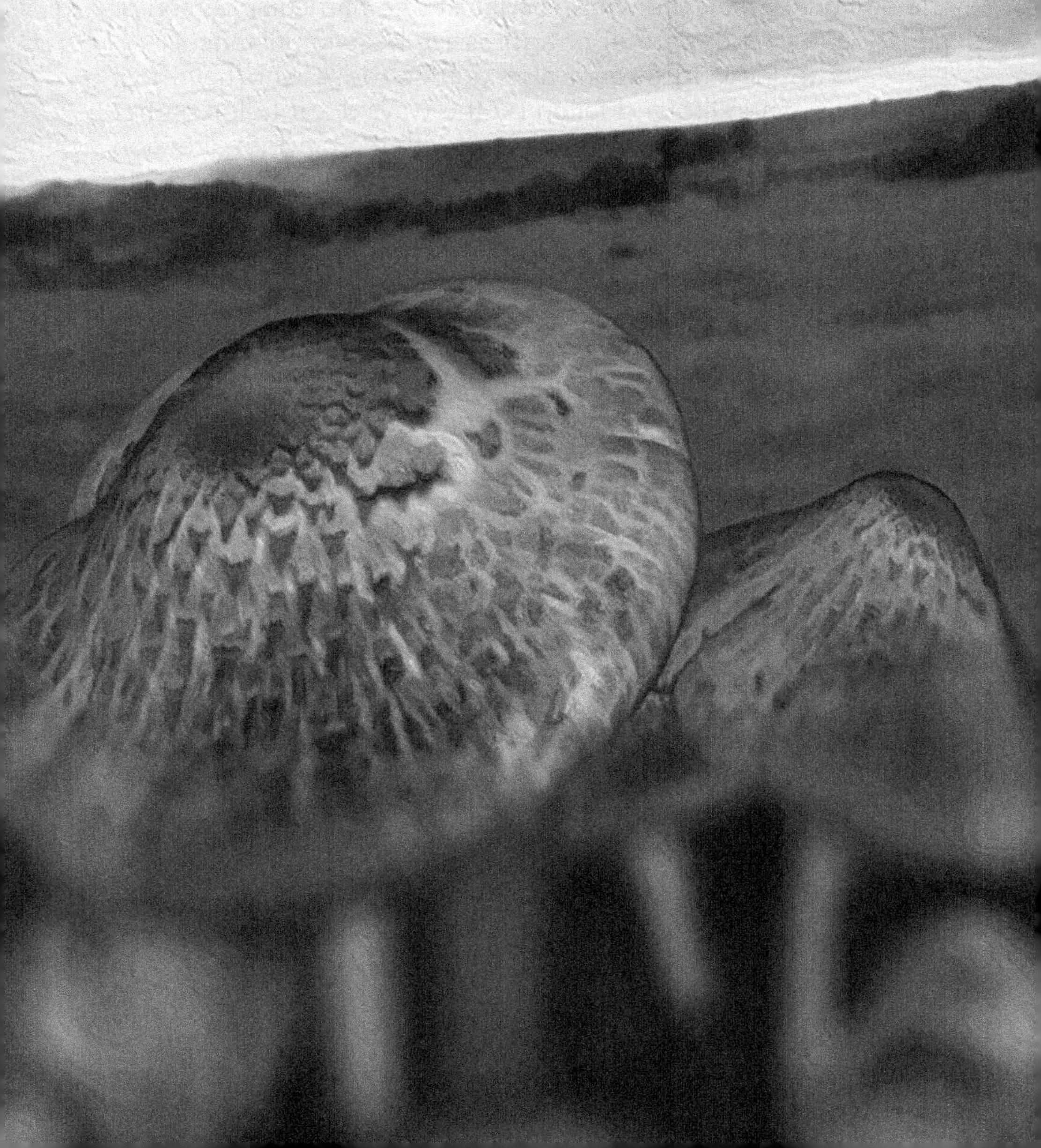

THE FLOWING STREAM

The stream constantly flows in a natural movement downhill, creating energy dynamics that are vibrant, yet focussed in one direction. The Flowing Stream is thus an excellent choice for those who require Celtic Reiki treatments with a directional intent – so you can use the essences as a way to focus on a particular issue or area.

Examples of this could be using Coll, Phagos and Nuin in a Stream Treatment for somebody who is facing impending exams or maybe Luis, Tinne, Duir and Onn for those who require the ability to assert themselves against one particular person or situation (a violent partner or aggressive boss for instance).

The Flowing Stream also guides those who have lost their direction in life and fallen by the wayside. It helps gather momentum, but in a specific way, not with the random direction and dynamics of Air. The Water always flows towards the sea. In this respect the Sea becomes the goal, the stream is the path and the Celtic Reiki essences are the boat in which you travel.

Excellent for use in manifestation treatments, particularly where the manifestation is a state of mind, health or emotional state: examples of these could be 'Inner Peace', 'Joy', 'Abundance', 'Healthy', 'Rested', 'Enlightened', etc. You can also use The Flowing Stream for the fluid systems of the body such as the circulatory or lymphatic systems.

Technique:

1. Begin with your preferred method of entering Core State and connection to the Wise One Mystic.
2. Internally state that this is to be a "Flowing Stream Treatment".
3. Stand at your subject's head with your hands at their temples and activate your chosen tree prescription either as a Treatment Forest or in the Woodhenge.
4. Once you have a definite feeling of energy, just relax and let the energy build, experiencing the essences of Celtic Reiki throughout your body. Start to become the energy, allowing the potency of Dwr to well up through the base of your spine, through your lower

abdomen, shoulders, then let it cascade down through your arms. Remember to keep 'soft knees' during this entire treatment.

5. When you are ready, start to move around your subject, as and when you intuit, all the time maintaining this level of energy – you are the stream, flowing through your subject, washing away their pain, focusing their energy, enabling them to flow with you.

6. Complete this treatment, going with the flow for an hour, or as long as you think is necessary to attain the intent of the session.

7. At the end of the treatment, create the final head connection with your client by placing your hands, lightly on their temples. Thank the Wise One for their assistance and then work through any usual closing routine that you have.

8. Bring your subject into the room, make sure they are lucid, and then offer them some water to drink.

Of Earth and Stone

This magical, Father Earth based technique is grounding, yet it does not necessarily work by grounding the subject—I have found it is more likely to ground the Celtic Reiki treatment with the client, thus having a more integral affect.

So this could suggest that when treating somebody who is overly grounded, you could work with a 'head' orientated tree, such as Saille or Gort and use Of Earth and Stone to ground those essences within your client. This would not ground them any further, but would instead lift them to a deeply grounded but 'lighter' energy.

As with The Flowing Stream, this technique is excellent for manifestation purposes, except here the focus is on material or physical manifestation, such as finances, property, a home, a soul mate, more time, etc. I have also perceived this treatment as very beneficial to the supportive structures of the body such as the skeletal and muscular systems as well as all the internal organs.

With use of the Standing Stones and their connection to the earth and past, this method can be used not only for physically-centred treatments and magic, but for yielding wonderful results in connecting to the past, both karmic and ancestral. Thus you can deal with past life issues and with disease or trauma that has been suffered by a person's relatives and by humanity in the wider sense.

So, if you know your client's grandmother died of heart failure, you could use Gort (heart), Ioho (Death) and Of Earth and Stone to clear the dynamic that caused this death —I believe this means that there is less chance of your client succumbing to this vibrational 'miasm'. You could do this on the wider picture too, for example using Luis (Immune System), Tinne (Sexual Disease), Coll (Boosts Physical/Emotional Healing) and Sycamore (Acceptance) to help ease the world of the HIV/AIDS pandemic.

Technique:

1. Initiate the treatment with your favoured method of entering Core State and connecting to the Wise One Mystic and make a connection with your client.

2. Now state with your inner voice that this is to be an "Of Earth and Stone Treatment".

3. Stand at the head area of your client, with your hands at their temples and activate your chosen essences of the Woodland or Standing Stones Realms either as a Woodhenge or a Stonehenge.

4. When you can feel the Celtic Reiki essences, just relax and let the energy build and take your attention to your subject's feet at the opposite end of the treatment couch. Visualise a pillar of Pridd essence rising up to the same height as you are, just below your subject's feet. Then see two more pillars rise up, one at either side of your subject (at '3 o'clock' and '9 o'clock').

5. Then visualise eight more pillars of Pridd, in between the existing pillars and you, so that you have a circle of standing stones that look like the face of a clock (if you were to be looking down from the ceiling). Now feel the Pridd energy rise up through your feet, completing the circle, as you become the 12th standing stone.

6. Now spend between 3-5 minutes at each point in the standing stone circle and as you stand at the location of each stone, place your hands on, or above your client – you may find the circle is elongated, like an oval, but this does not matter.

7. At the end of the treatment, make a final head connection by placing your hands gently on or either side of your client's temples, thank the Wise One Mystic and then work through any usual closing routine that you have.

8. As with all treatments, ask your client to come back into the room, make sure they are lucid, and then offer them some water to drink.

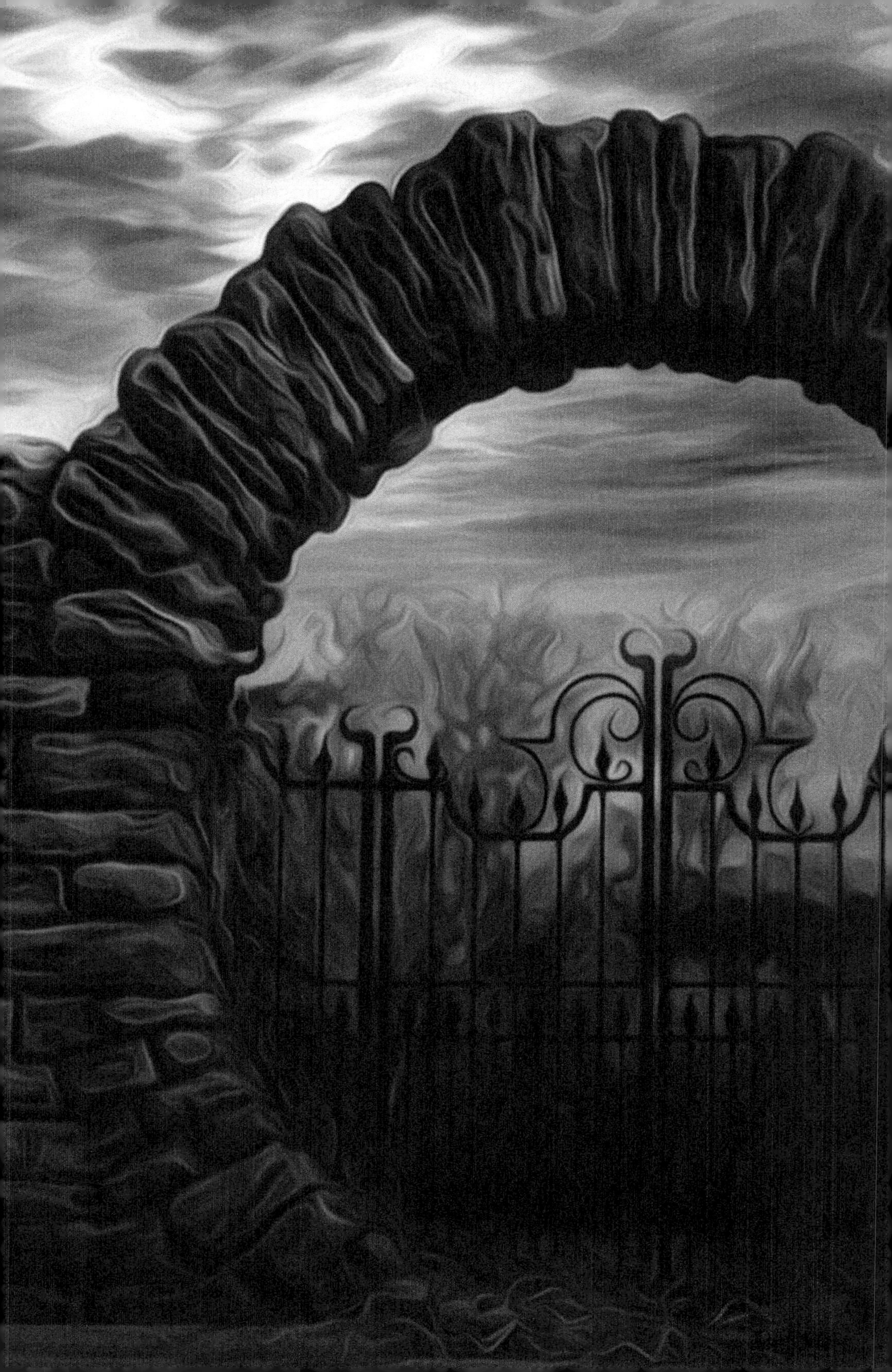

A Wise Choice...

There are times when every Mystic faces tough decisions and needs to trust in some greater force at work. The Mystic that knows each challenge and what some might deem to be 'failure' represents an opportunity that is far beyond our conscious understanding.

It was one of these occasions that she pondered as she returned from the shop where she had connected to the man. She battled the limiting beliefs that had been instilled in her life; beliefs that nudged her in the direction of pity, of despair, and of viewing this man as tragic.

It was a final glimpse of some possible future that she had witnessed as he left, some choice that had been made, which chilled her to the core. She had watched him leave the store and out of her life; though the last image she had seen within her mind was one of a man, curled up in his favourite chair waiting for death.

This death did not come in the grasp of some dis-ease, but by the hand of another. She felt the presence of death behind him, as he sat staring from the window, she experienced a spectral hand around his throat, squeezing the life from him, and she knew with everything that she was, that he would soon reach the end of this life at that final meeting.

The Wise One had reconciled the conundrum of death and rebirth a long time ago. For any forming of healing is a death and rebirth - a transformation from dis-ease to ease. It is a common belief that the path to healing is one of life, however, in this complex dance, any action taken creates the transcendence and therefore death of the old.

She understood that the important role for her in this situation was not only to heal her own challenges and underlying pain, but also to offer whatever support she could to the man from the shop, albeit at a distance. In a world where every person has a choice, it was clear to her that her role in life was to support the choices of other people, even when those choices differed from her own, or even when she disagreed with those choices.

Every moment is a moment of the now. Be it a current

experience, a memory or a visualisation of some future date. When you reminisce, you are doing it in the present, when you dream of things to come, you are doing so in the now.

What we label 'the past' and 'the present', are merely a difference of encoding in our minds. Some aspect of a thought is recognised by the consciousness as being separate from us by time, another deception of perception. The Wise One knows that in every moment, something must change in order for us to be aware of the passage of time. Change means birth, it means death and it means the rebirth if this moment into something new.

The nature of choice is one that comes with its own complexity, as we are responsible for our own choices and all the consequences of those choices.

With each and every step, we create 'ripples' that expand out into the world and change everything. The conscious mind is very good at giving continuity and at filtering out certain chunks of information, so very often we are completely unaware of the results that we obtain through our choices.

The Wise One considers all choices with total responsibility for all consequences, expansive and contractive. Experience has taught the Wise One that, even though they are motivated by a sometimes selfless need to help others, when it comes to choices, one needs to do what is best for the self. This way we ensure the best we can give to others. Placing oneself into a situation where we give more than we can, leads to all manner of circumstances—usually those where there is a tendency to blame others.

When treating others, we often encounter intuitive responses that are upsetting or unwanted in some other way. These are mere possibilities and the Wise One knows that whilst their intuition is very accurate, we live in a Universe of infinite choice and every person can change their mind at any time. If they do so, everything changes. The Wise One trusts their intuition (how they define others), but they are also guided by people's right to turn from their current direction.

With this in mind, the Wise One makes decisions based upon their own healing agenda and needs. This Mystic will consider others needs to the utmost, yet their awareness of how basing important decisions on the fickleness of others can lead to having 'the rug pulled out from underneath their feet' if another person changes their mind, means that the Wise One ensures they are happy in themselves with each choice made.

At times, the Wise One encounters those who have made the choice to die or act in some way that is detrimental to wellbeing or destructive in a wider sense. When this occurs, the Mystic knows we cannot make them take another path; and nor would we want to, because this is all a part of greater perfection.

So, the Wise One simply does what they can to help—easing pain, minimising the effects of dis-ease, nurturing the qualities that can help each person find what they are searching for. By doing so, we complete our responsibilities to the client, without compromising ourselves in the process.

The Wise One Mystic is also very aware of how time is merely an illusion of perception - and that all thoughts are in the present, even if they are interpreted as the past or future. Therefore, to assist the Warrior Mystic in their role, the 'past' is seen as potential (not actual) and can be changed in our perception.

To support the Alchemist, the 'future' is also treated as the present, with an understand that 'what we want, but have not yet attained', is actually 'currently attained, but not yet recognised by the conscious mind'. This way manifestation is brought into the present and becomes a matter of recognition, instead of creation.

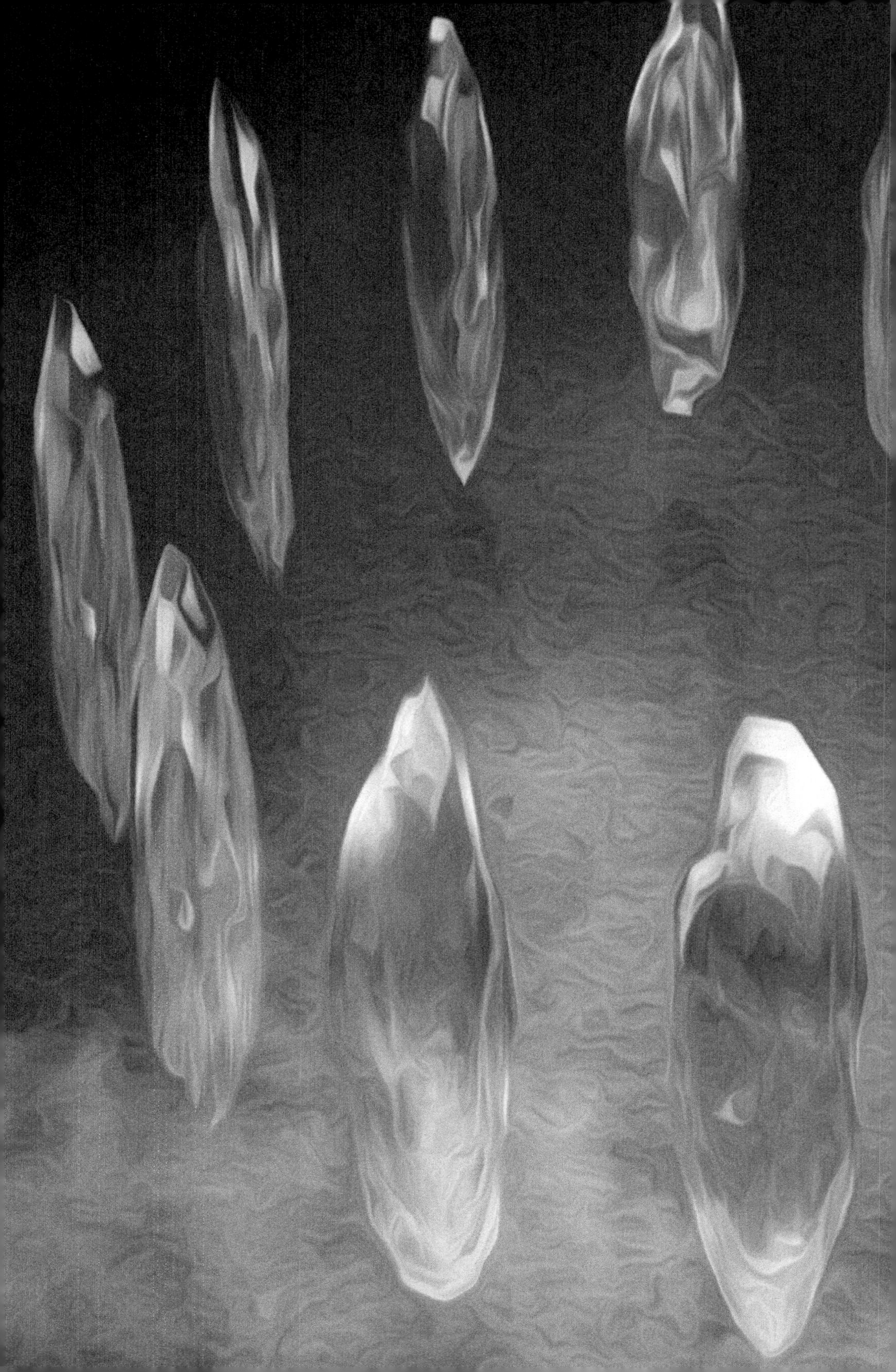

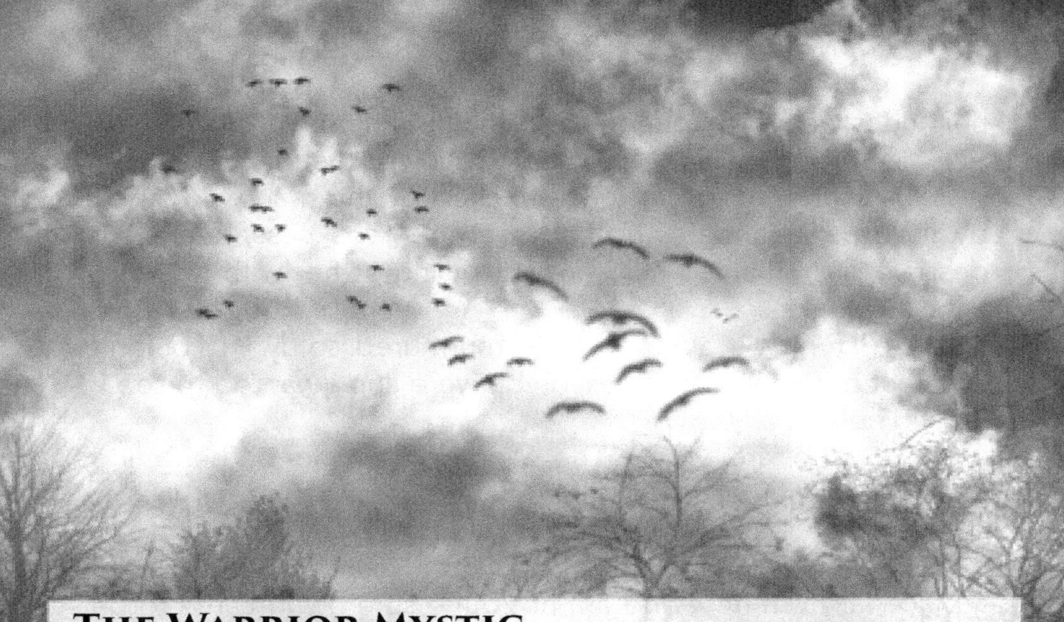

The Warrior Mystic

The Warrior made her way through the Woodland Realm, towards a stretch of open scrubland. Her mood was pensive that afternoon and as twilight came she found herself doubting her own abilities. It was as if the light was waning within her, as well as from the sky above. She was so wrapped up inside her introspection that she was by the ancient tree of Fearn before she brought herself back into full awareness.

Climbing the mound that led up to the ancient tree, she was stunned by the enchanting silhouette of the gnarled trunk and branches, set against the fire oranges and reds of dusk. The Warrior placed her hand on the trunk and sighed mournfully.

"I do not know what to do!" she exclaimed in the Fearn tongue. "I do not want to go to war, yet we are being terrorised and my people are looking to me to lead them!"

The tree listened with a kind and gentle demeanour, absorbing the words with such respect for their sacred nature that each syllable seemed to be plucked from the air and squirrelled away, inside the tree's very being. The Keeper of Secrets would never speak of the Warrior's concerns to any other, for he was the one that the strong go to when they feel weak; when those who cannot falter, falter and need a listening ear that will never give their secret away.

"I feel so completely lost!" She cried, as she slumped to her knees weeping, as a grieving child might weep.

"Please…" said an unfamiliar voice, "Let me help you."

She leapt to her feet, shocked by the man who stood by the tree; this man who had seen her weakness, heard her despair. He remained still, simply smiling at her with his kind, knowing smile.

"Don't be alarmed." He murmured softly. "I couldn't help but notice how distressed you were and I wanted to see if I could help in any way."

"Who are you?" The Warrior demanded, her mind quickly assessing all the different factors and options in this situation.

"I'm simply an adventurer on a journey. I come from a place far from here and am not quite sure how I came to be here. I really didn't believe I would ever find you." The man spoke truthfully and seemed very earnest in his gestures and body language.

"So you are not from this part of the Realm?" she asked with a sidelong stare.

"I'm not sure I'm from the Realm at all!" he exclaimed with a half-chuckle that seemed to be derived from bemusement more than anything else.

The Warrior relaxed a little, grinned and said, "Everybody comes from the Realm!"

The Warrior has inner-strength and confidence in his abilities. This does not mean that he cannot falter or feel lost on occasion, however, when he does feel the pang of confusion, he trusts in his ability to find his way through.

He knows with unwavering confidence that the answers are near, that he is equipped with everything he needs to discover them, and is strong in the knowledge that at some point, things will change.

The Warrior takes full responsibility for themselves and their life. They never blame others, no matter how challenging it is to be completely accepting of all that has happened, without exception.

This Mystic will share his issues with others, but is always careful not to say things that damage his self-esteem or define greater challenges; he understands that to think it is to bring it nearer and to speak it is to make it physical.

Whereas the Wise One uses action and ritual to conduct treatments and practices, the Warrior is more introspective; using thought and emotion to attain the things he sets out to achieve. Hence, there is very little 'externally-based' methodology in the Warrior's art—his skill exists with his internal power and how he 'frames' himself consciously.

Although the Alchemist is the most cerebral of all the Mystics, the Warrior does use an internal voice as his compass, yet this is emotionally-centred and internal, as distinct from the higher-mental activities of the Warrior.

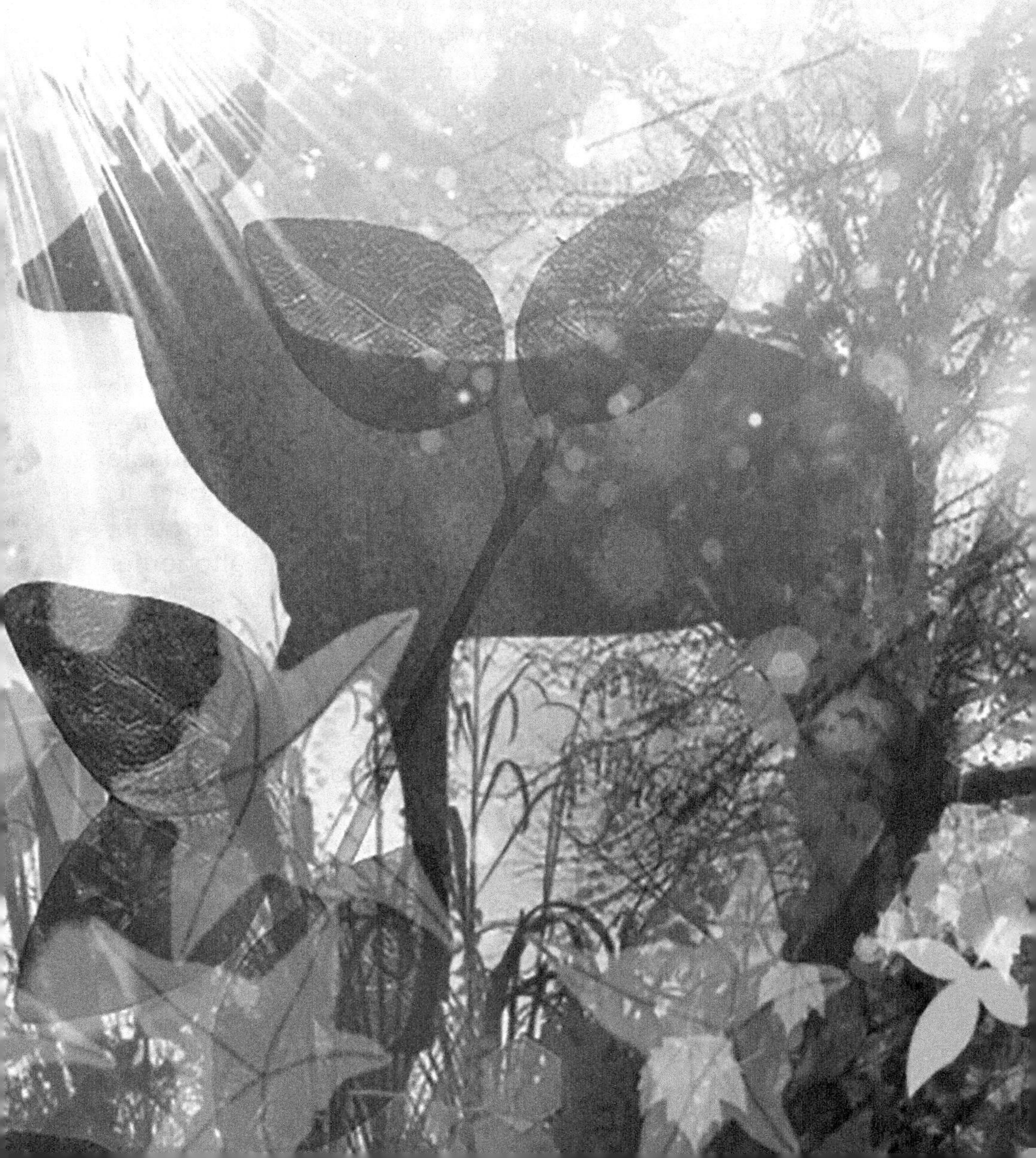

Connecting to the Warrior

We live in a society, where many are trained into feeling out of control. We are born, we hope for the best, we have a destiny, we are lucky/unlucky, we get sick, and we die. This is our life, our world and very rarely do we question this, because most of the time we believe it to be true.

When we look around our world, we have been trained to perceive evidence of this that compounds our belief that we exist at the whim of some seemingly random force. From how bad things happen to people, to the way that good things happen to people, we regularly witness hurt, war, dis-ease, miracles and people winning the lottery. Each day we are subject to occurrences that prove life is something that happens to us.

Once in a while somebody will try to tell us that this is not the way it is, we may laugh at them for suggesting such quackery, or we may listen to what they say, then try to do what they suggest in order to change our world. We may experience failure, think "what a waste of time" and yet, something inside is saying, "This is not the way things are, there is something more to life than what you perceive there to be!"

This is the voice of the Warrior Mystic; the perspective that constantly anchors a strong, self-assured, powerful inner-voice into your world. At times when you feel you lost or unable to persevere, the Warrior Mystic consistently pulls you back to your path. Even when you are saturated with doubt, frustration, or anger, the Warrior is courage, confidence and is altogether sassy.

When you first connect to the Warrior Mystic, you may notice how your conscious focus shifts so that you notice more positive reenforcement of how you affect your life. Whereas you could have previously 'filtered out' instances of self-realisation, the Warrior will proactively direct your attention to examples of your own power.

This is accompanied by a real sense of self-assurance, high esteem and assertiveness. If one is usually plagued by an inner-monologue that is critical and naysaying, this will slip into the background; swept away as the volume rises on your innate talents and abilities.

The apparent difference between the connection technique that you encountered earlier, for the Wise One, and that of Warrior Mystic is an emphasis on your emotions. The Wise One is focused on layers which exist on more spiritual/less physical areas of consciousness.

This requires the enactment of specific, physical rituals that replicate non-physical actions, in the physical world. (Think back to the shaping techniques and how you enacted the creation of a triangle to represent energy that acts like a triangle.)These actions are a 'statement of intent'; an external mirror of what is occurring internally at expanded levels.

The Warrior is centred to a greater degree on your physical being and your emotional-self, so hand movements, breathing and other ritualistic actions are replaced by introspection, perception, and the monitoring of how you feel. Here the ability to coordinate mental visualisations with physical movements is swapped with a need to calm your thoughts and focus solely on your perception; be it emotional, sensory, or synaesthetic.

For many, this may seem more elementary to complete than the often complex array of steps that are involved with spiritual ritual. However, the art of stemming the incessant flow of internal monologue and the habitual thought-patterns that vie for your conscious attention can take much practice!

It is for this reason, the Warrior Mystic invites you to develop a mastery of your mind, because this not only helps you clear a space to acknowledge your emotions over the 'noise', it also prepares you to master your emotions with thought and conscious affirmation - a skill very few people actually learn.

Some people view the mastery of thought over emotion to be calculating and cold, yet this is not the case. We can indeed halt the explosion of anger in an argument, or stifle the urge to 'bitch' about the things or people that frustrate us.

Conversely, the very same ability can also stop any thoughts from interfering with the complete enjoyment of a quiet, blissful moment and enable us to commit absolutely to love, joy and rapture.

Technique:

1. As with the Wise One Connection, start the process by sitting or standing in a suitable position, making sure your spine is upright, shoulders back, neck and head

are aligned with your body and that you are facing straight ahead. Keep your arms and legs uncrossed, and if standing, have your feet a shoulder-width apart and your knees 'soft'.

2. Focus on your breathing, by taking your attention to the effect of breath on the sides of your diaphragm, just below the ribcage and on your abdomen. The in-breath should cause you to expand out the sides and your tummy to rise. The out-breath contracts your sides and tummy, whilst you pull your lower abdominal muscles inwards (and when you are skilled, inwards and upwards). With each breath, count from the number one, upwards, trying to increase the count with each breath. Remember that the exhalation count should always be greater than the inhalation.

3. When you feel very relaxed and your mind is still, affirm internally that this is to be a "connection to the Warrior Mystic" and then you enter Core State, although instead of visualising an 'internal star' as you have done previously; practice entering Core State based on emotional response alone. In other words, keep you mind blank and focus only on the sensations and feeling as you approach your Core Self. This may take repetition and you will need a clear understanding of the Core State visualisation before attempting this variation.

4. In Core State, keep your mind disconnected from any thoughts and direct your attention solely to your feelings. Concentrate on simply being for a moment and then, locate the Warrior Mystic simply as an emotion, sensation or 'gut-feeling'.

5. Move this feeling towards you, keeping all else at bay and avoid paying attention to any other thoughts or emotions that attempt to block you or limit you in any way. Focus only on the 'Warrior sensation' whenever these distractions attempt to turn you away from the task at hand.

6. Finally, connect to the feeling and embrace your

Warrior self. Experience the world in as much sensory depth as you can and ensure that you connect into the emotions as much as you can. It may take several attempts to master this technique and on occasion you may need to reacquaint yourself with the Wise One Mystic before working with the Warrior; though it will eventually become very easy and possibly instantaneous to achieve.

7. When you are ready to disconnect, simply thank the Warrior and feel yourself transitioning into your usual-self.

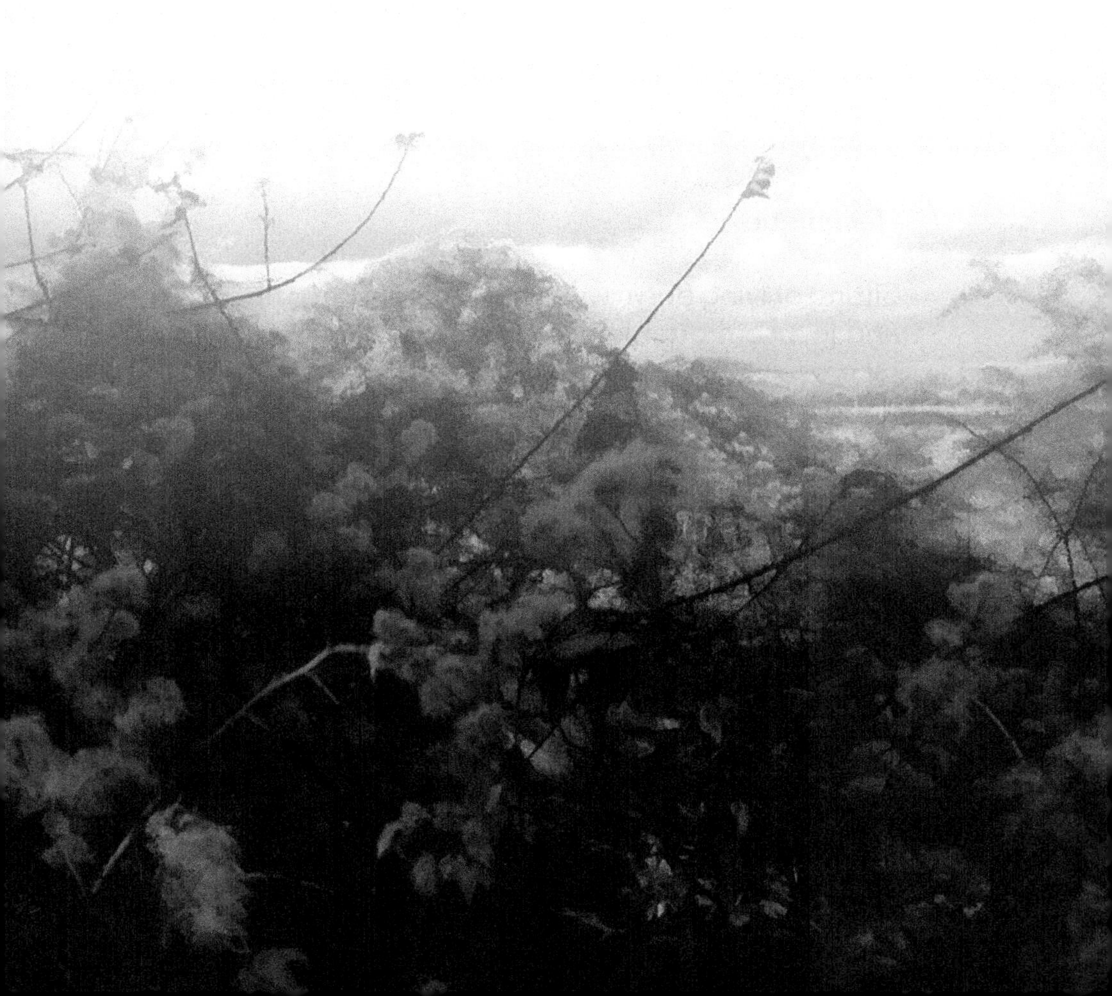

Realm Shifting with The Warrior

The underlying processes of Realm Shifting in the Warrior perspective are almost identical to those of the Wise One Mystic.

Nevertheless, the emotional/spiritual contrast between these two, also carries over to the way we conduct the Realm Shifting process. Here the technique has an integral focus on the sensation of shifting, as opposed to ritual and internal statement. Hence we achieve a richer, sensory experience that affects our Realm Shifting abilities overall.

Some find they prefer one way of shifting between Realms over others and have a tendency to stick to their favoured method. Whilst this is perfectly adequate for practice, the exploration of all Realm Shifting styles, has a layering effect that creates a mastery of process on all levels; physical, emotional, spiritual and cerebral.

You are therefore, encouraged to plan your Realm Shifting, so that you maintain a fitting style for each practice you conduct: when treating a client, use the Wise One method; when building confidence, the Warrior style; and if you are studying, work with the process described in the Adventurer's Guide (p. 113).

Technique:

1. Sitting or lying down with your arms and legs uncrossed and in a comfortable position, with your back straight, take your attention to your breathing. Take several deep breaths into your lower back and abdomen, using the same style of slow, regular breath as you have done with the previous exercises.

2. With each exhalation, find yourself expanding and on every in-breath, 'fall' into yourself – not downwards, but inwards, as if flying to the centre or core of your being.

3. Internally, say that you are entering "Avatar State" and repeat the mantra "Warrior", three times, or use your favoured trigger method.

4. Feel the internal shifting from 'you', to 'you as the Mystic, Warrior'. Wait a few moments for this to occur

then proceed.

5. Choose the first realm you want to work with – such as the Furthest Ocean, for instance—and internally, ask the Warrior for this to happen. Focus on your emotion and feel a shifting take place, internally - this could be emotion, sensation or synaesthesia-based.

6. Once you have entered the realm, use your emotions to hone in on the nuances of the realm. Become attracted by expansive, joyous emotion, whilst filtering out contractive feelings.

7. Once you have discovered your optimum realm experience, explain to the Warrior Mystic that you want to go to the next realm (stating your second realm choice by name, for example, the Woodland Realm).

8. As you shift, be absolutely aware of any sensations, synaesthetic reactions and notable experiences that you can use to recreate this transition at a later date.

9. Once you have completed this for all five realms, come back into your conscious awareness of your physical environment and, when you are fully awake and focused, make notes on your experiences.

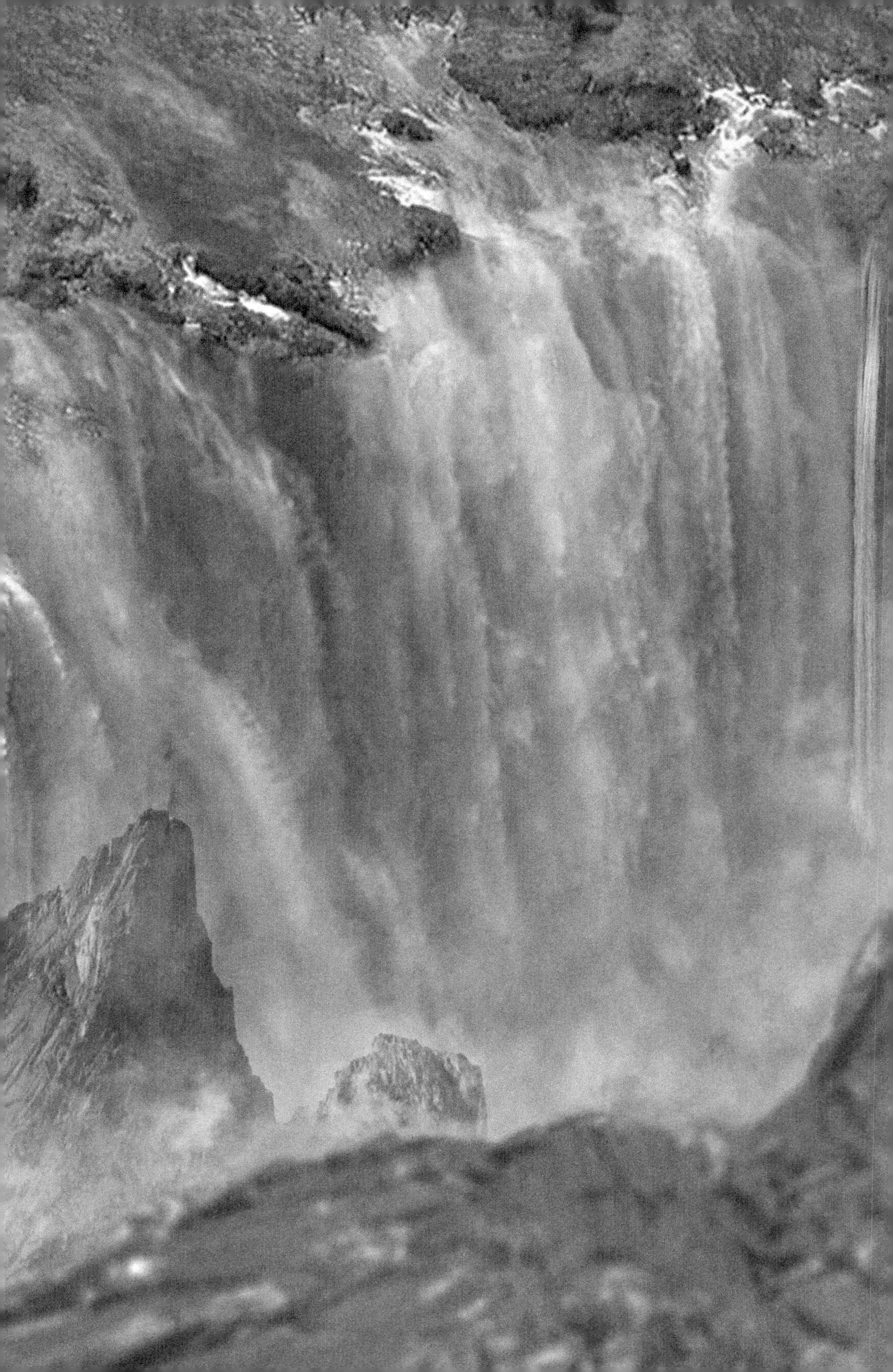

THE CALM BEFORE THE STORM...

From that day onwards, she would return to the tree on the mount, meeting the stranger from a faraway place. They seemed to be so different, so unlike each other, yet this did not stop them from falling in love. He would speak to her about things beyond her understanding and she would share the tales from her life.

More than this, though, she was able to be herself with him; not some facade or fiction, used to impress others. She felt strong, whilst being permitted to be vulnerable without diminishing that strength. For a stone has nothing to defend - it is strong throughout. It is those who are fragile within that are the most courageous, for they have guardianship of a most precious gift.

For the briefest time, she was able to forget the approaching storm that would eventually present her with a difficult decision. This was not an avoidance of her responsibility, but a chance to experience joy, despite what may come. For the Warrior has the ability to laugh when it is time to laugh, no matter what sadness exists around the corner.

The Warrior negates worry through planning and foresight. She knows that contemplation of a thing, gives that thing power, so if a future event may be painful, why waste happy moments thinking about what might be. Conversely, she was about to speed the transition of challenging times, through a deliberate focus on joyous occasions to come - not existing in some far off future, but available to her now.

Hence, she spent long days, lying in the shade of the tree, talking with the stranger. Every moment, falling in love, relishing the experience of finding connection with another. She cherished every moment, though she could never touch the man, never hold his hands or kiss his lips. To do so would break the spell that brought them together and he would return to his world, never to be seen again.

And as the autumn came, the red-tainted horizon of dusk foretold of the battle to come. The Warrior knew the time had come to face her final battle and regardless of how little hope there was of her returning, she used her fear to make her stronger and experienced her love more than ever; knowing if anything would bring her home, it was what she valued the most.

It was in the late afternoon, when the leaves on the trees were turning to rust and umber that she heard word that the fearsome army of invaders had arrived and it was time to defend her people. As she made her way to the tree for what could be the last time she saw her love, she made it her mission to get through this war, so that she might be with him again and that they could hold each other close.

She found him standing under the tree, smiling as she approached - he knew nothing of her challenge to come and this was how she wanted it.

For his smile lifted her up, for the expansion of others helps us to expand, even when we feel lost. They stayed together until dark, until it was time to part. As they bade each other farewell, she told him she would see him again soon, and though her heart was breaking within her chest, she walked away with a bold stride and joy in her step.

The Warrior knows that we experience expansion and contraction, as these are both essential parts of life. The experience of the physical world is not one to be lived in constant, never-ending bliss, nor is it intended to be shrouded in darkness, locked away from bliss and kindness.

The Warrior would not have it any other way, because he knows that in times of contraction, we give contrast to our own wonder and perfection. This contrast enables us to reach beyond ourselves and experience the gut-wrenching happiness that only comes from knowing some other place.

The way of the Warrior Mystic, is to use the contraction to the utmost of his ability, so that the times of expansion are even greater. So, he lives in every moment; soaking up the joy and using it when hardship comes.

He surrounds himself with pro-active, supportive and encouraging people and ensures that he mirrors these attributes back. This way, when we find ourselves troubled by circumstance, the words and actions of those around us keep us buoyant and afloat on the roughest seas.

The Warrior also ensure that if ever he feels a pang of concern or worry that he takes some action to rectify this. Rather than sitting around, wrapping himself further into a conundrum or getting caught up in contractive thought patterns that spiral into unhelpful emotions, he will actively change his behaviour and alter his thoughts with those that produce the feelings associated with wellbeing and contentment.

He expresses gratitude for all he has and cherishes the things that have made him who he is, regardless of what he sacrificed because of those things.

As a fiercely emotional creature, the Warrior Mystic does not shy away from the depth of his feelings; he simply knows how to use emotion in a proactive way - to achieve goals and emerge victorious... even when the outcome may appear to be the complete opposite.

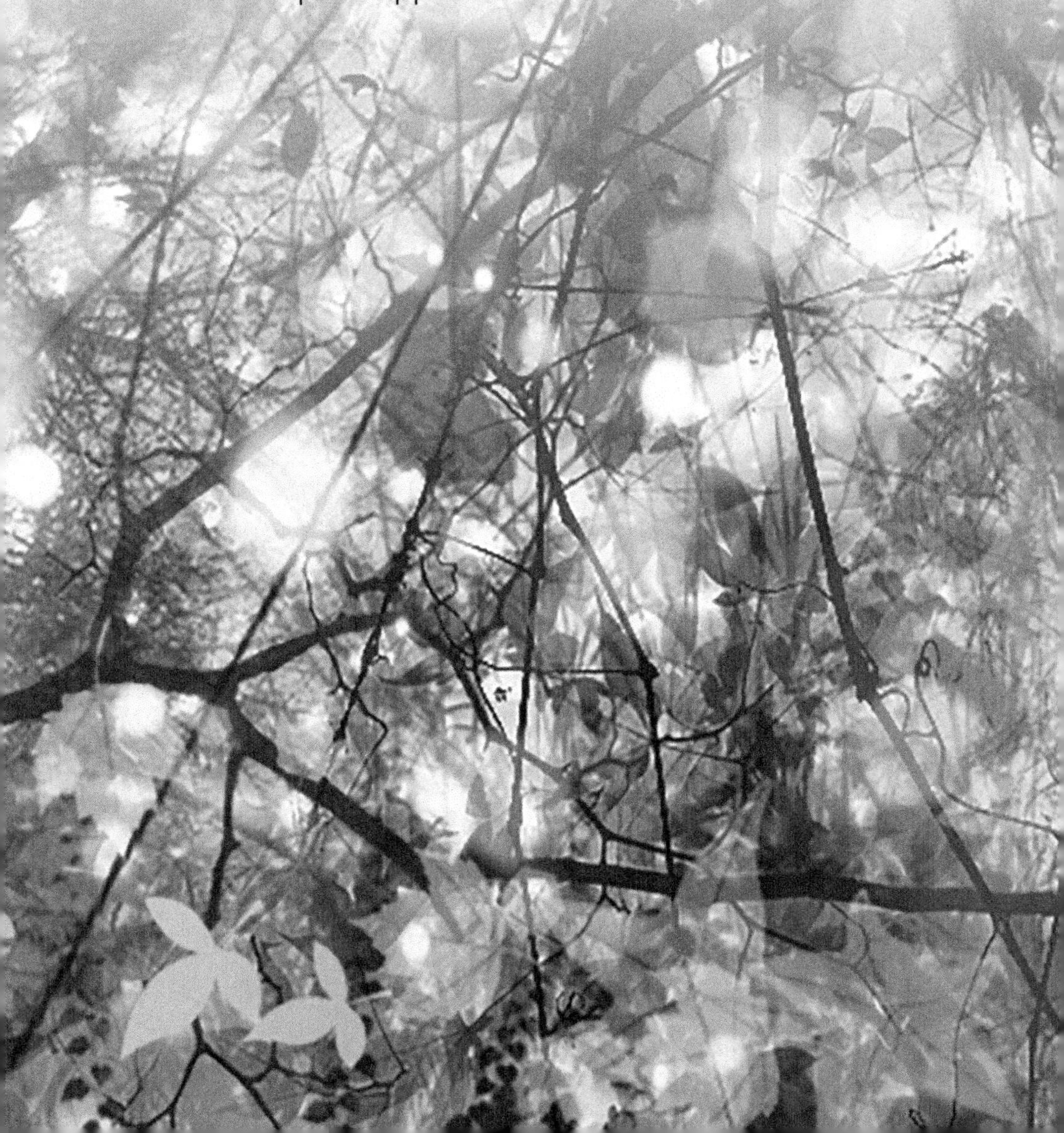

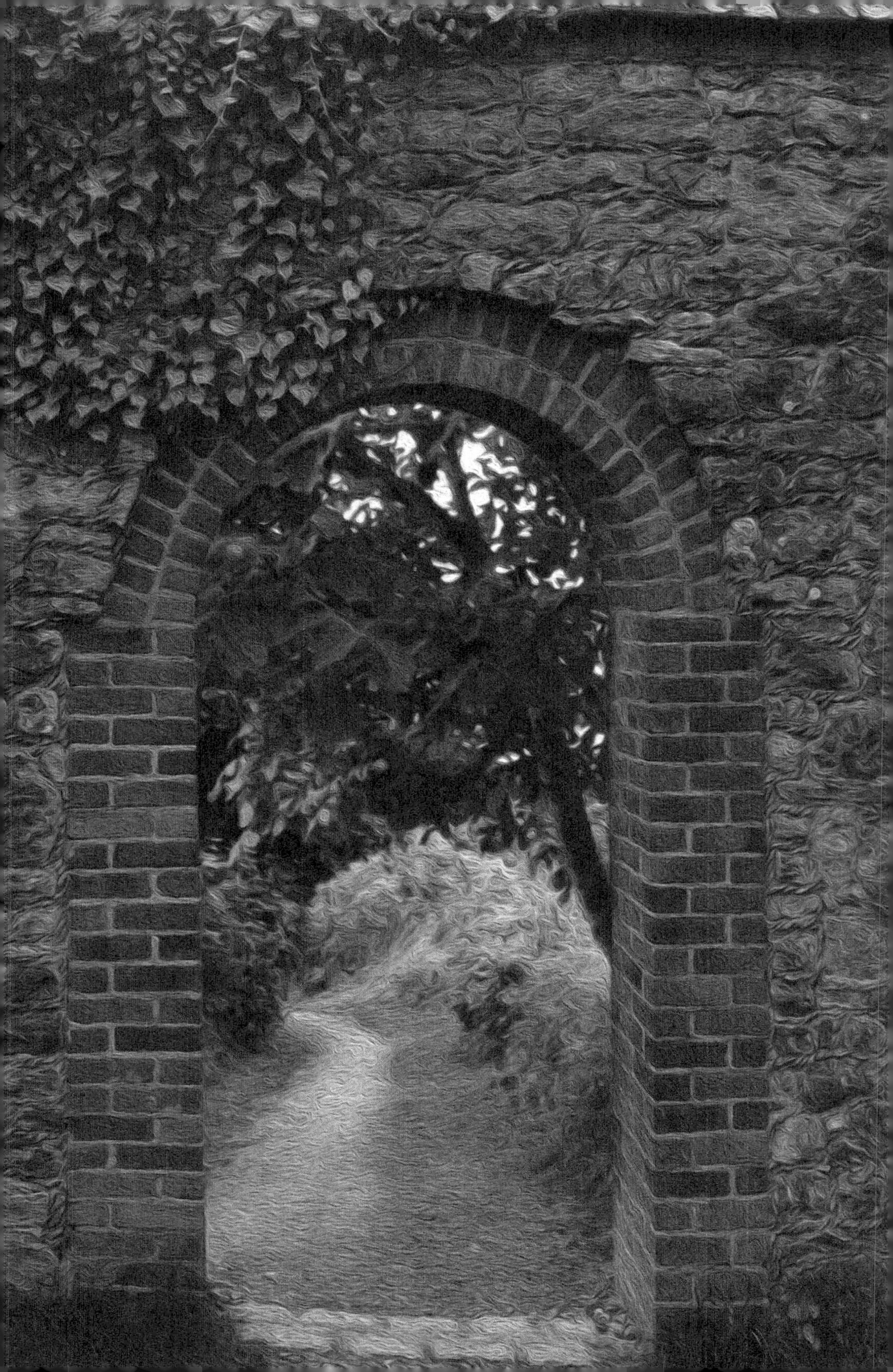

Development Methods of the Warrior

LlynFawr (Clin-vower)

Llynfawr is a method that the Warrior can use to cultivate Ki or Nearth, which is a progression from 'The Ki & Nearth Potential Technique' used by the Adventurer Mystic. The word LlynFawr translates to 'The Great Lake' and is symbolic of the reservoir, or the place where Ki is stored in Eastern philosophy: the Dantien.

Technique:

1. Sit in a comfortable position, relax your body and mind, close your eyes, ensure that your spine is straight and that you are comfortable with good back support. Your feet should be placed firmly on the floor and your hands should be positioned palms down on your lap. Now take your attention down to the lower abdomen, around 3 to 5 centimetres below your belly button, and really explore the sensations there while affirming to yourself internally that you are about to do LlynFawr.

2. Place your right hand on your left collarbone, with the palm flat against your chest then, in one continuous motion, bring your hand down across your chest and down to the right hip. Do the same motion, but using your left hand on the right shoulder. Complete this stage by repeating the first motion, beginning with right hand on left shoulder.

3. Using the right hand, stroke from the left wrist across the palm and out past the fingers of the left hand. Do this movement again reversing your hands (left hand brushing right hand) and then repeat the original action (right hand brushing left hand).

4. With your hands raised high in the air, palms upwards and fingers pointing directly behind you, connect to the essences of Celtic Reiki. You can do this by

visualising the essences as light surging down into your palms, flowing down your arms and into your body, at the same time pull essences up through your feet. As you become aware of the sensations you may feel your arms begin to lower. If you do not feel this, start to lower them anyway. Bring your arms out to the sides 'pulling' the essences around you as if you are creating a bubble around you. Bring the energy/light down past your head and up through your legs, into your body, holding it in your abdomen. Then pull your arms down and around to meet on your lap, palms facing the stomach and your dominant hand closer to the skin.

5. With your hands still on your lap, palms positioned towards your body, focus on the essences that are there. Now place your tongue against the roof of your mouth just behind the top set of teeth and contract the perineum. Breathe in deeply; drawing air into your lower back and allow your stomach to rise and your chest to expand to the sides. Visualise energy flooding in through your crown and feet, through to your abdomen, gathering there with each in-breath.

6. Now, as you exhale, allow your tongue to fall, relax your perineum and feel the energy flowing out from your abdomen, travelling vigorously from your palms and fingers, your feet and toes. Then repeat the process by inhaling as you did above. You can continue with this technique as long as you like, or is comfortable for you. However, if you begin to feel light headed or faint, stop immediately. This technique should be used with caution by those with high blood pressure or in the latter stages of pregnancy.

7. The next stage is achieved by placing your hands together as if praying and positioned just above the heart centre. A good way of checking if you have the right positioning of the hands is to gently breathe out through the nose, you should be able to feel the breath on your fingertips. Whilst maintaining this position, remember to breathe as in stage 6 unless the

contraindications already stated suggest otherwise.

8. Become aware of the place between your middle fingertips. Focus on that space and completely clear your mind of all else. You may find this challenging at first but as each new thought comes into your awareness, just acknowledge it and send it away very calmly then bring your attention back to the place where your middle fingers touch. The more you do this, the more you will learn to just 'be': not only a valuable state for Celtic Reiki practice, but also an incredible state for spiritual enlightenment.

Entrainment Styles

The art of entrainment is when one body 'entrains' another to the same 'state'. This could pertain to a happy person entraining a group of depressed people to an elevated mood, or a mobile phone set to vibrate, causing a harmonic 'rattle' in the desk it is resting upon.

When used in Celtic Reiki, the term entrainment denotes a way of creating a change in some environment, be it a physical location or the 'environment of the self' (the combined and holistic states of oneself, including every facet that is defined as being connected to the self). This change brings the environment to the intended perspective of the Warrior.

Healing treatments are also a form of entrainment. In the viewpoint of the Warrior Mystic, we use entrainment to specify that we are working environmentally, rather than personally. This is a vital distinction, because a treatment of oneself or others targets an individual directly—when you entrain the environment, you are filtering your Celtic Reiki through the 'environment of you'.

A useful analogy here would be working with a goldfish in a tank; a healing treatment would target the fish, whereas an environmental entrainment would treat the water. However, in practice, you are not directly treating the 'room' or place you are at—you are entraining your perception of/connection to/influence over the situation or circumstances of that place and the people in it. (If a Master focused solely on the water surrounding the goldfish, would the results differ if she held the intent of making the water of better quality, rather than making the fish more healthy?)

The first practice we shall examine here is a technique for entraining a contractive environment—usually a physical location or area that either feels detrimental to the wellbeing of those at that location or causes some unwanted response. When faced with these places, you may also wish to conduct a self-treatment after this routine, to ascertain exactly why you are reacting towards the environment and heal any 'wider' effects.

Technique:

1. Describe what it is about the environment that is causing the issue, thinking carefully about the words you use: oppressive, draining, stressful, over-exciting, stagnant, etc. Then think of an essence that would change this, so for example: sunlight, the Atlantic Ocean, Koad, Yellow, Tinne, and so on. Pay particular attention to what feels good, as you intuit your essence(s).

2. Once you have your chosen perspective, start the treatment by standing in the environment and focusing inwards.

3. Scan your environment; be aware of it, not only in the physical sense, but energetically, vibrationally, perceptively, and so on. Get as much sensation as you can and monitor this closely as it occurs.

4. If you feel exceptionally contractive at any point, hold the sensation and trigger your preselected essence(s). Notice if this quashes the contraction and if it does, this is a best essence for the task at hand. If not, intuit other essences, until you shift from the contractive influences.

5. Once this is done, search beyond the present moment and physical location you are in. Explore every instance of the contraction, past or future, nearby or at any physical location.

6. Now shift every perspective to that of your essence(s),

constantly monitoring your emotions and synaesthesia responses to adjust and hone your entrainment of the environment.

7. Thank the Warrior Mystic and come right back into your conscious awareness.

The Warrior Mystic will urge you to take full responsibility for any contraction you encounter - even when it seems as though it is the actions of others that are causing the contraction. To this end, the following technique helps to alter the 'environment of a situation' and enable you to empower yourself in creating change; even in the actions of others.

Instances of the environment you might want to tackle are: debt/lack of finances, structural/physical problems with your home, business difficulties, unsuitable job, loneliness, etc.

Technique:

1. Isolate the challenge you are letting go and then locate the underlying issues, for example, debt may be down to your feeling unworthy of abundance, or an unsuitable job could be the limiting belief that you have to be unhappy in your work. Remember to ask yourself – If I have 100% accountability, why would I choose this?

2. Scan everything you understand to be defined as 'you', in as much detail as you can. Include your physical body from large systems (circulatory, muscles, etc.) to the smallest building blocks (visualise your cells, DNA, and atomic structure). Follow your emotional and mental journeys, recognising feelings and thoughts, but not connecting to them. Remember to keep your focus on the task at hand. As you encounter the areas that are connected to your current situation, hold these in your awareness, until you have a 'layered stack' of issues.

3. Hold this 'stack' at a location where you can maintain awareness of it, but still continue with your scanning.

4. Then repeat the scanning, except on this occasion, monitor your body, emotions and thoughts for points where this challenge does not exist - areas that feel really peaceful, vibrant or energised. These are the regions of your being that appear to be in a different reality from the challenge, as if completely unconnected.

5. Stack these expansive elements and hold the two stacks side by side in your mind. How do each of these feel? How could you make the contractive stack feel like the positive stack? What essences could you use?

6. Prescribe the essences that you decide upon, to the contractive stack and continue enveloping every part of the stack until you feel it shifting perspective toward the essences.

7. As you feel the shift gathering momentum, reassert your expansive stack as a template and then follow every single link the contractive stack has to other areas of your being. So you are not only treating the challenge, but heading away from the challenge to treat all the dynamics and sources that created the challenge in the first place.

8. When the contractive stack and its associated areas of your being feel more like the expansive stack, come back into the physical environment and fully return to consciousness.

Technique:

This is a fascinating style of entrainment, because even though the challenge seems completely unconnected to you, you still treat the environment of 'you' (Imagine everything you know as 'I' to be an environment in which your consciousness lives).

This will have a profound effect on the way the other person or situation acts after you have completed the technique. This can be startling, especially when you treat an issue that you have no involvement with (or feel you cannot affect). For instance: a conflict on the other side of the world, or a trauma that a friend has experienced.

1. Discover the root of the 'external' issue within yourself; for example, relationship issues, actions of others towards a loved-one, a legal dispute that is affecting a client, a famine, natural disaster, environmental issue, etc. Where are you responsible for causing this situation—even if it is just 'thinking about it' or 'directing energy to it' - time is energy and if you spend time thinking about a challenge, you are converting 'time-energy' to a source of power for the challenge!

2. Scan your entire being and define any aspect of yourself that is empowering the challenge's ability to exist in your perspective. As in the previous exercise, stack these parts of yourself and hold in your awareness.

3. Next, work with the process from the previous exercise [4], by locating the expansive layers of your being. These are facets of your being that seem completely removed from the challenge in definition and feeling.

4. Hold the two stacks side by side in your mind and compare them. Intuit what essences, shapes, etc. you could use to treat the stack and everything it is linked to.

5. Prescribe these resources to your contractive stack, until it matches the common themes of the expansive stack. Whilst you are doing this, monitor your emotions, thoughts, etc. Add any thoughts or emotions that present themselves as you are treating to the appropriate stack.

6. Once you have completed this, come fully back into the room and your waking consciousness.

THE DYNAMIC WARRIOR

Throughout our Celtic Reiki Adventure, we have examined the notion of contraction and expansion as a means of differentiating between what many would call 'negative' and 'positive' experiences. Negative means less than zero and positive means more an zero.

What we usually mean when referring to something perceived as 'negative' is 'not nice' or 'detrimental to wellbeing' and so on. However, 'negative energy' literally means 'less than no energy' - energy that is detrimental to wellbeing or not nice is still energy and exists in the positive side of the scale. A negative experience is still an experience (positive), no matter how 'not nice' or detrimental to wellbeing it was.

In the wider context, no experience, energy, circumstance is negative or positive, good or bad, nice or not nice - it is simply experience, energy, circumstance. In a universal context, the way of things just is - it is our emotional attachments that create the sensation of nice/not nice, etc.

A millionaire could look at the life of one with no money and decide this was a negative experience. Equally, the happy pauper could view the miserable, but ever-so-wealthy person and decide that it is far more positive to be poor.

Good and bad are contextual, even though we all know what each means to us. When we think in terms of good/bad or positive/negative we place ourselves at a disadvantage. For example: how many broken hearts fill the subconscious mind of a person who links their happiness with finding true love? When a businessman has an underlying belief that successful people have 'horrible personalities', how would this affect their business?

The emotion of good/bad, positive/negative is very definite and creates decisive responses within us. The definition of good/bad, positive/negative changes from person to person, is vague, based on context and leaves us second-guessing and sabotaging ourselves at every turn.

Traditionally, the concept of spiritual growth has also been viewed with this 'two-point' principle - you ascend or descend - go up, go down, there is good, there is bad (evil), and so on. These concepts have a real value in some contexts - when you are surrounded by 'evil', focusing on good can help you survive. Yet, in the somewhat sophisticated society of the West, we have moved beyond the notion of traditions in so many ways that a modern perspective is needed to develop our spiritual evolution.

There is such an atmosphere of 'the real world', where people believe only what they can 'see' or 'touch' (even though seeing and touching is more likely to throw up illusion than 'knowing') that we need to appease this in order to evolve spiritually.

Remember, even though you may consciously 'know' what you know - if you are aware of anybody (even one person) who does not know what you know, they represent a part of your being that needs a more advanced way of being spiritual.

Another challenge with the up/down model is that you can only ever go 'higher' or 'lower' than you have been before. There is hardly any scope for other considerations. For instance, you ascend further than you have ever been, you can descend further than before also!

The lessons you learn today help you get 'so high', but what happens when future lessons negate this one? Does this mean you deny future lessons or have to completely change your viewpoint? (Think about the brouhaha caused by the Theory of Evolution and what it meant for the Judaeo-Christian understanding of Genesis.)

Therefore, the concept of expansion/contraction provides us with a greater level of sophistication, whilst preserving the semblance of a two-point philosophy. When you expand (like a balloon), you do so in every direction and you become less 'dense' or less 'physical' in nature.

Contraction creates density and physicality - you become more solid. This illustrates how spiritual growth is a choice, not a coercion. There is nothing detrimental or bad about contracting into the physical world to enjoy the experience it holds. It is equally joyous to expand into source and to create experiences of bliss and enlightenment.

The 'spherical model' of perspective and perception has revolutionised Celtic Reiki and personal-development systems like it. The understanding that perceptual movement in one direction creates identical movement overall is an evolutionary step forward. We 'solidify' and 'etherify', according to our choices and there is no rebuke or punishment for either; just freedom to be.

Everything you have ever done and all that you know can be embraced by the spherical ideal - even if you have had to completely reconsider your beliefs and attitudes at some point, there is wholeness in the sphere that enables contrasting and conflicting ideals to be at peace with each other. Every part of the sphere has a different perspective, externally and internally. Some points exist, directly opposing each other, but neither is right or wrong, they just do their part in the creation of the whole.

A major consequence of this from a Celtic Reiki perspective is that our move into history—beyond the philosophies of Usui Reiki—has pushed us forward in knowledge, higher in consciousness, deeper in integrity, further in creativity, increased our logical understanding, and given us a much wider scope of practice. Our system may not be as 'dense' as Usui Reiki, yet this presents us with the flexibility to make Celtic Reiki our own.

As we expand our 'awareness' (knowledge, consciousness, understanding, etc.) of our art, there is the possibility of becoming so expansive that we lose physicality and cohesion in our beliefs. This is often seen when people are ridiculed or seen as having mental illness for their beliefs. Of course, this is contextual, for any hint of something spiritual is seen as 'weird' by some. The important factor here is that your rate of expansion remains cohesive, tangible and solid enough for you and your clients.

If you find your thoughts, experiences and rationale becoming disjointed or seemingly fragmented from the rest of your world, the Warrior Mystic can bring greater 'density' to your spherical perspective, without creating contraction. This is an absolutely remarkable ability, because it means that you can regulate your spiritual growth by expanding at your own pace and strengthening that expansion with a denser volume of awareness.

At anytime you may choose to contract into physicality to: help others; to experience some physically-based activity and 'be completely in the moment'; or simply because you want to spend time with the physical body. The act of contracting never diminishes your expansion—it is purely experiential contraction (as is your expansion).

Technique:

1. Sit or lie down in a comfortable position that maintains the natural alignment of your spine, neck and head. Keep your shoulders relaxed and back, arms and legs crossed, close your eyes, and focus on your breathing.

2. Take several, long breaths, bring air deeply into your lower lungs and blow the air from your body in ever-increasing lengths of exhalation. You should feel as if you are expanding to the sides, back and front with each inhalation; rather like a balloon.

3. Shift into your Core State, working with the Warrior method for shifting and spend a few moments here, relaxing and preparing for the expansion.

4. Now return your attention to your breathing and use the breath to create a definite sensation of expansion and contraction in your physical body.

5. Gradually, feel that your physical environment is expanding and contracting with your breath. As you breathe in, the room or place moves nearer towards you. As you exhale the physical environment expands.

6. Extend this contraction and expansion to beyond your immediate surrounds, see the earth, trees, creatures, sky, sun, planets, stars, cities, people, etc. All expanding and contracting with you.

7. Now select an essence that symbolises 'strength' to you—perhaps Duir, Clear Quartz, Sequoia, or the colour Red. Project this outwards as you exhale and hold the level of contraction as you breathe in.

8. Now breathe out once again and continue the expansion from where you left off. Continue this until the expansion is as far away from you as you can visualise.

9. Find yourself completely filling this 'space' and then bring the sensation of this expansion, fully back into your waking awareness.

Tip for the Warrior

There may be occasions when you wish to contract into the physical reality of another person—to help, support or communicate with them. Usually people trigger a contractive emotion to do this - anger, aggression, frustration, etc. However, the 'chemical-backwash' from this, makes it challenging to expand again and therefore jeopardises the intent of the contraction.

You can use this technique to contract, without emotional-chemical responses, by reversing the expansing/exhalation in steps [7] and [8] to contracting the essence with inhalation. So, inhale and contract the essence towards you. Hold the essence at this level as you breathe out and then begin the contraction, once again, with the in-breath.

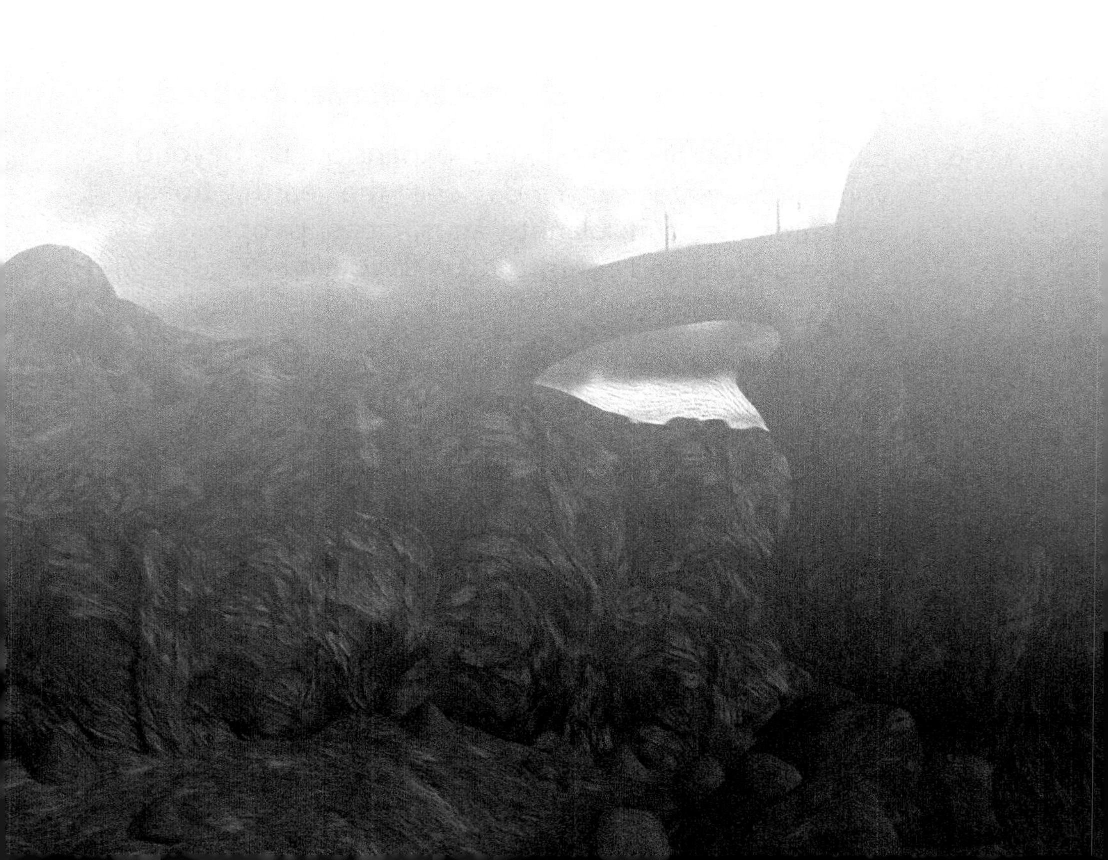

Intuition Enhancement

Just as the healing perspective is integral to every aspect of Celtic Reiki, intuition and psychic ability are engrained within every Mystic; each having their own particular use for these arts. The Wise One intuits the best healing method and essences for their client's wellbeing, the Adventurer knows which path to explore, and the Alchemist perceives endless results and combinations in the mysterious regions of CosmicLore.

The Warrior is the only Mystic to have these abilities for their own sake. The prophetic wisdom of the Warrior is matched only by their ability to decipher the unknown or more precisely the 'what cannot be known'!

The Warrior interprets like no other, using metaphor and symbolism where no words exist. They perceive the enigmatic realms of synaesthesia and inner 'sight' in incomprehensible detail and translate these for other to understand.

To achieve the level of connection, in Avatar State, to the Warrior Mystic for these abilities to be awe-inspiring, you will need to practice. This technique can help you master your Avatar State and the ability to intuit via a connection to the Warrior Mystic.

Technique:

1. Stand in the centre of a room, in a quiet place where you will not be disturbed for the duration of the technique. Centre yourself, close your eyes, and bring your attention inwards. Turn your attention completely to your breathing, taking long, slow, deep breaths that cause your stomach to expand and chest to move outwards to the sides. Breathe this way until you start to feel relaxed and very calm – if you feel dizzy or light-headed, sit down for a while until you feel better.

2. Place your hands out in front of you, palms facing down, and push downwards through the air until you reach a resistance. 'Sit' your hands on this cushion of energy and relax your arms into this resting place.

3. Ask the Warrior to create sensations and feeling

that you can interpret and wait for a response. This response should take the form of a slight 'magnetic' pull in your hands which should direct one, or both, of your hands to the left/right. You may also find this sensation pulling you forward or back and do be prepared for this with your 'soft knees'. If the pull takes you beyond the comfortable reach of your arms, you can walk slowly in the desired direction.

4. Now search for changes in movements of your hands and continue to explore these changes until you find dynamics so 'heavy' that you cannot push through it without using muscle effort. Bounce your hands along this dynamic, until you have a good idea of the boundaries. Then push your hands further into the dynamic – if the force is too strong and pushes you back, or resists completely, push your fingertips of your left hand into the barrier, creating a claw with your hand that pierces the energy, as opposed to pushing.

5. Once you have done this, ask, in your mind what 'this' is and then clear your mind as best you can. Allow images, words, feelings, sounds and so on, to fill your mind. You may find it helps at this point to clarify what you perceive by speaking your experiences aloud.

6. Upon completing this, come fully back into the room, have a seat and take a moment to compose yourself and make any notes.

Craiddseren (Cried-thser-ren)

This technique can be used to increase your intuitive or psychic awareness, enabling you to achieve more accuracy in readings, treatment or manifestation techniques. In Celtic Reiki terms, the word 'psychic' does not pertain to ghosts and the supernatural, but rather an ability to know what cannot be known in relation to the wellbeing of ourselves and our clients.

Technique:

1. Sit in a comfortable chair with your feet firmly flat on the floor, your spine straight and your head up. If you wish to play some gentle music, light candles and burn essential oils, this will help create the right ambience required for the exercise.
2. Take a few deep breaths and relax, attempting to release any tension that you are holding. Feel yourself sinking back into the chair yet maintain your straight spine and head up position.
3. Now take your attention to your forehead, lifting your eyes to look at the centre of your forehead, under the closed lids. Keeping this eye position take six slow, deep breaths, each breath lasting six seconds on the inhalation and ten seconds as you exhale. If you cannot do this, take twelve breaths of three seconds for each inhalation and five seconds for each exhalation. With each breath, feel yourself lifting upwards as if you are stretching towards the ceiling of the room.
4. Now place your tongue to the roof of your mouth, just behind the teeth and contract the Perineum. Relax your eyes while continuing to keep them closed. Activate the Celtic Reiki Essences of your choice.
5. Now imagine that you are looking into your head and all is dark except for a small point in the centre of your head. You might want to imagine this point as a star or as a ball of energy. As you travel towards the light, you want to hone in on the most central point of your

head, so that as you get closer, the point becomes smaller and smaller.

6. Maintain this visualisation for several minutes. If at any time during the exercise you feel as if you are falling backwards, go with the sensation and just allow yourself to float 'head over heels' repeatedly.

7. Eventually you reach the central point and bathe in the light. As you just float here in the light, start to immerse yourself in the essences, visualising them all around you, beginning with your hands, feet, head and then travel into the centre of your body. When you are completely immersed in essences, get a real sense of how this feels.

8. Now start to nurture the sense, there is a bubble of Celtic Reiki all around you and this bubble contains all the infinite patterns and dynamics that exist from the perspective of these essences and their source trees, minerals, etc. Start to see these 'unwrapping', as if you are shedding the surface layers away to reveal what is hidden underneath. Start off with one or two individual dynamics (which you could see as threads or lengths of string, maybe even as 'energy onions') and then start to simultaneously unwrap all the dynamics at once, seeing the 'peelings' fall away from you. As you do this, the light gets brighter and brighter; the Reiki more and more powerful.

9. Floating at the centre of your head, unwrapping all the essence dynamics, start to be aware of every single thread/onion/dynamic in existence. Feel each one extending from this central point outwards into the infinite Universe – never-ending, always flowing. Start to expand outwards along each and every dynamic – reading it, knowing it. Make sure that you expand equally in all directions; taking your time at first to ensure that you are increasing the size of the energy bubble in a uniform way, then becoming faster and faster. Decipher every dynamic equally and at the same time – do not focus on any one dynamic.

10. Continue with this until you recognise the motion/sensation created by travelling along the dynamics and can simply flow with this feeling without thinking about it. Continue this for as long as you wish and then come back into the room.

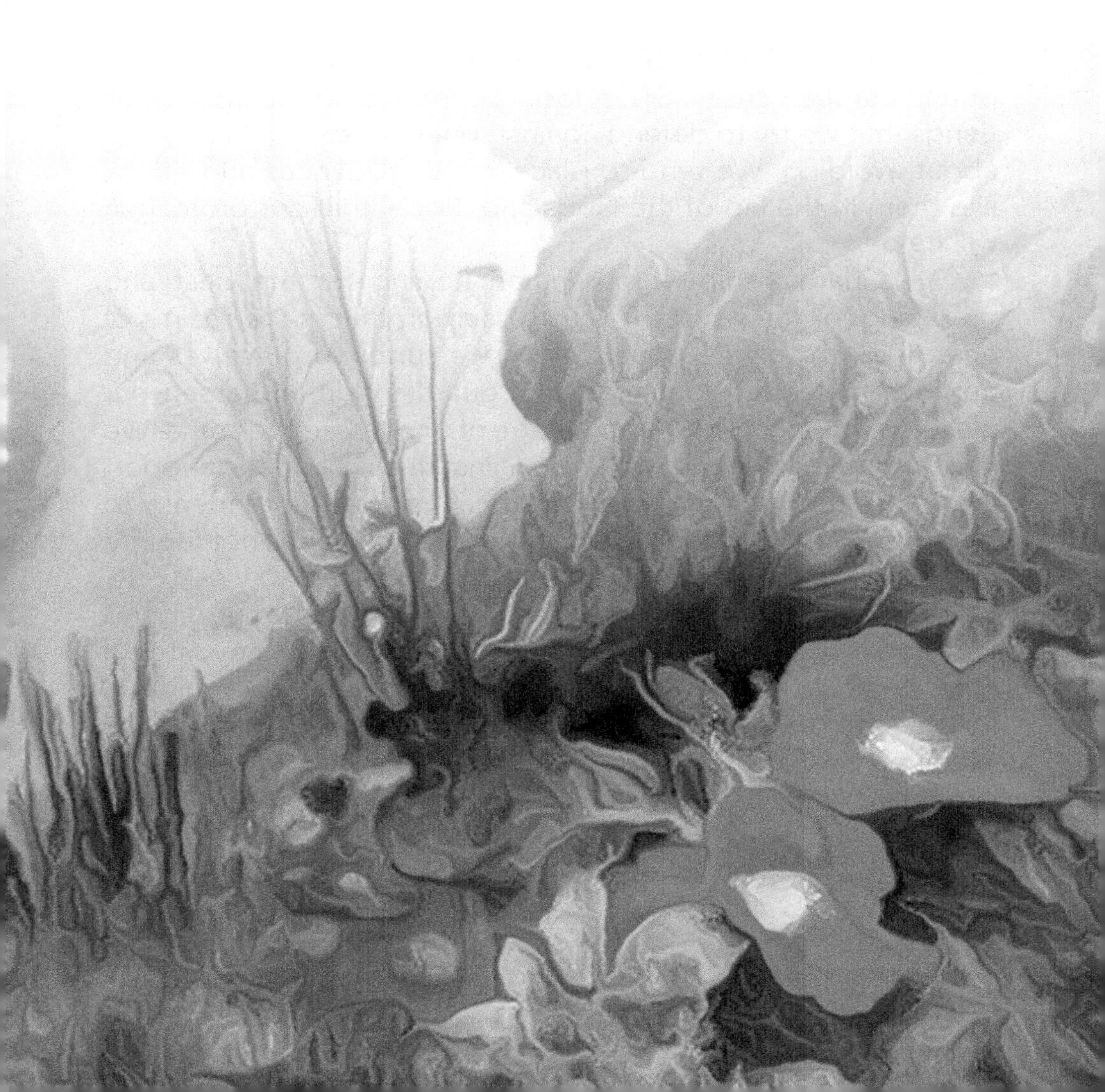

The Warrior Guardianship

What many describe as 'protection', the art of the guardian is to preserve that which is in their care. To assert oneself, maintain boundaries, and stand strong in the face of challenge all uphold the notion of 'protection', without one, unnecessary, inclusion.

Psychologically, we attach significant meaning to words—a word can conjure up all sorts of emotion, depending on the connections we have previously formed with that word. For many, the word 'protection' has 'positive' connotations, however, we only ever 'protect' ourselves against things that are intangible, unknown, or in some way 'bigger than us'.

We protect ourselves against dis-ease, against accident, against disaster, against the weather, and so on. Terms such as 'unprotected sex', 'payment protection insurance', 'protect and serve', and 'anti-theft protection', all conjure up thoughts of uncontrolled crises. STDs, losing one's job, and crime are all things that we try to defend against, but ultimately feel helpless about avoiding. We tend to place these incidences and others like them in the lap of the Gods and 'hope' that our protection will help.

Guardianship is more than hoping for the best and preparing for the worst - it is the assertion that in the realms of energy, all things are equal. When we surround ourselves and our loved ones with boundaries of guardianship and assert our place, we bring the inner-knowledge of oneness to the arena. We understand that we only defend against the self and the support the self is attempting to provide. So, if you have a tendency to subconsciously sabotage your best efforts, this does not require protection; it needs understanding and resolving.

The Warrior provides the strength to stand our ground and look the issue directly 'in the eye'. Thus, we are offered time to really explore the challenge, when usually we would run for cover at the mere mention of it. This understanding in itself will often lead to resolution, or, at the very least, suggest how a conducive conclusion can be obtained.

Technique:

1. Stand upright and centred, with your feet firmly on the floor, a shoulder-width apart, your spine straight and head up. Shoulders nice and relaxed.

2. Shift into Core State, using the Warrior style of feeling-based shifting. Whilst you are doing this, breathe deeply and expand to the sides with each breath, exhale by blowing the breath as far away from your body as you can.

3. Create a low tone in the very centre of your head. You can practice this by making the lowest hum you can, so that it is easy to imagine. You could also use one of the low-resonance tree or stone essences of your choosing. (We all feel the essences differently, so you will need to discover which essence are experienced as 'low' for you personally.)

4. Start to raise the pitch of this resonance, making it higher and higher, whilst expanding in all directions to match the level of pitch. Go through the mid-tones and onwards to very high-pitched sounds. Continue until the sound, if an actual note, would be just audible and hold the pitch there.

5. Using your inner vision, 'ripple' this sound outward, like ripples in a pond, but in every direction—fill the physical location, circumstances, situation or other focus entirely with this sound.

6. Finally, come completely back into waking consciousness.

Tip for the Warrior

If you wish, you can also use one of the Celtic Tree Essence guardians to complete this technique, for example: Tinne or Luis. You may also decide to use a Standing Stones essence, such as Obsidian, Plutonium, Salt, Jet, Iron or Silver; or for a 'softer' effect, Schumann.

Confidence Patterning

Confidence is an essential part of Practitionership and Mastery of Celtic Reiki. The knowledge that you can achieve the results that you and your clients want and the strength to face challenges or obstacles is paramount to your professional abilities. Very often in training of this kind, a lot of consideration is given to treatment techniques, client care, ritual, and labelling, though very little is mentioned about the traits you will rely on to support these other elements.

Most people come to Celtic Reiki Mastery training with a deep-rooted compassion and desire to help others, some want to fulfil a need through healing or personal-development, others desire positive feedback or want to make a difference. You can probably resonate with all of these to some degree.

What is not so certain about those perusing a Celtic Reiki career is how able and comfortable they feel with the many different layers of practice and mastery. Cool-headedness, lateral- and unconventional-thinking styles are valuable, as is the ability to be an aggressive listener. In addition to these, confidence - in one's own skills and in Celtic Reiki - is vital. Without this, getting the results you and your clients deserve can be challenging.

Much of your confidence will stem from your training - your grasp of the Celtic Reiki methodology, that you trust your Celtic Reiki Master, the teaching materials, and the results you attain whilst practicing. The personal and external experience of your Adventure will also reflect on your confidence. There will be times when you feel full of confidence and others when you're not so sure. With a good foundation in place, this technique will enable you to work through the Warrior Mystic to grow your level of confidence and offer a much needed boost, if ever you feel a tinge of doubt.

Technique:

1. Stand with your feet firmly on the floor a shoulder-width apart, your spine straight and your head up. Keep your shoulders nice and relaxed.

2. To enhance the effect of this technique, place your

tongue to the roof of your mouth and produce a slight contraction (lifting) of your pelvic floor muscles (this is known as a 'Perineum Connection' and is used in many of the meridian-based therapies of Eastern Medicine).

3. With your 'inner vision', feel yourself falling forwards, as if you are tumbling towards the ground, yet remaining absolutely grounded and upright in physical body. Travel through the floor and back up again, in a complete circle, so that you end up returning to 'centre', through your back/back of the head. Repeat this several times, gaining a good 'rhythm' or 'flow', and speed up the rate of the rotation, to make it as fast as you can.

4. Trigger the essence or essences that currently have the most expansive or joyous effects for you. Carry the sensations created by the essence with you on your rotation.

5. Connect to the essence as integrally as you can, and then continue for as long as feels comfortable.

6. When you are ready, come to rest at the centre position, take a moment to attain a real sense of how you feel and then extend your right arm out, in front of your body, palm upwards.

7. Direct the sense or perspective of the essence(s) to the inner area of your elbow region (the place where syringes are used during the taking of blood). Keep this going for around 3 minutes.

8. Next, repeat this direction of focus with the left arm outstretched and palm facing up.

9. Place both hands on the centre of your ribcage and project your attention to the spine in the corresponding area. Do this for 3-5 minutes, maintaining your focus throughout.

10. Come fully back into your physical environment.

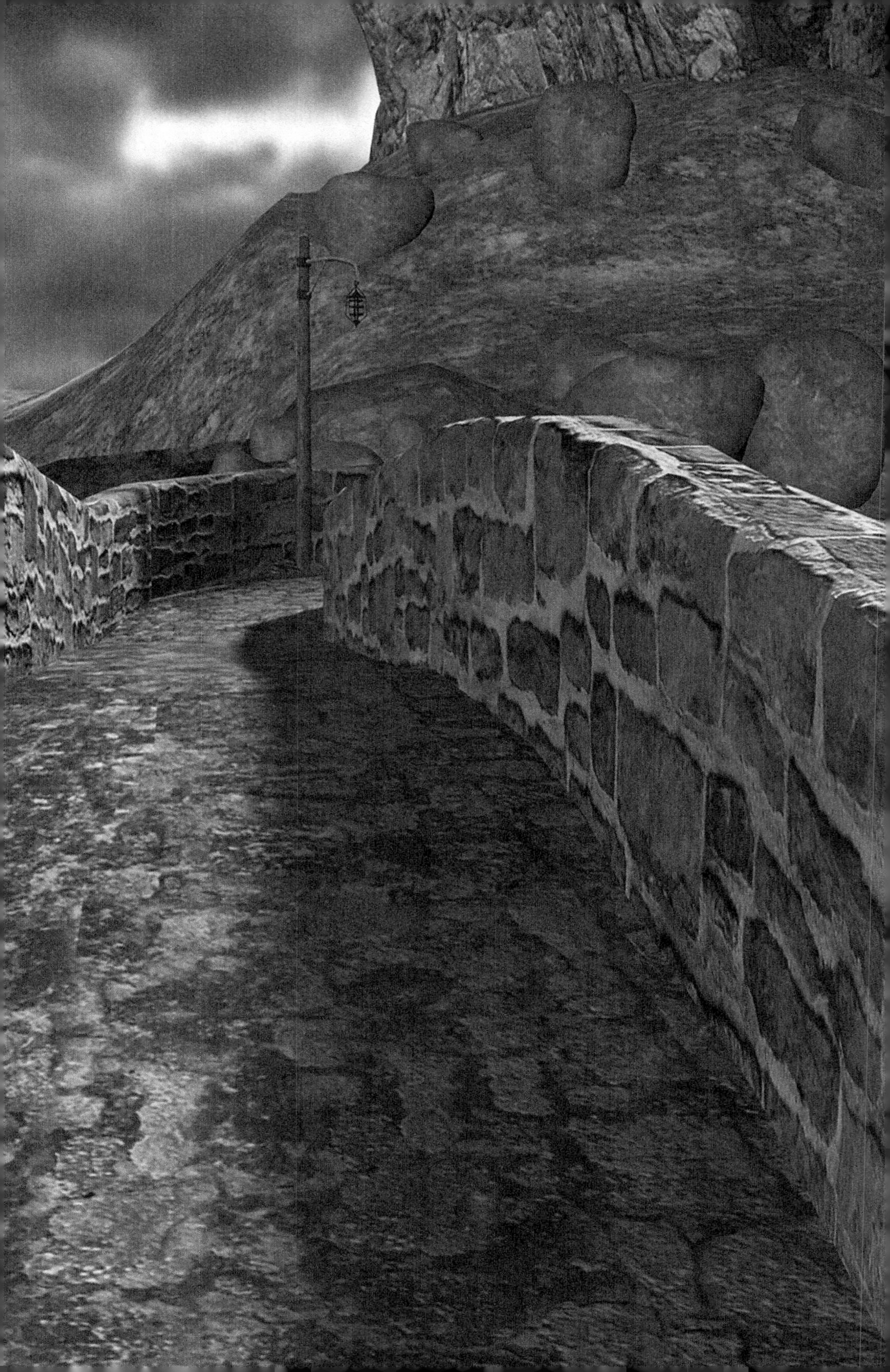

THE BATTLE BEGINS...

The charcoal grey storm clouds beckoned to her across the wide fields, toward the vast army that spilled over the horizon as far as she could see. Her step was of one unafraid, her head stared straight towards the challenge ahead and she inspired those who followed her with a charismatic air.

She had spent her life as a guardian of her people and was confident in her ability to lead others. What we do regularly and are experienced in gets easier, until there is no trepidation.

Today, however, she faced a force, unlike anything she had ever seen or known before. Now was a time to rely on her training; to do what she had learnt to do and trust that she was capable of holding back an incomprehensible foe. Of course, this is the nature of the Warrior Mystic—one who is prepared by experience or through training, so that when the skills are needed, they have a foundation to carry them forward.

In the chaotic battle that followed, no wisdom, training, or preparation could have made up for the sheer numbers of the opposing army that swept across the fields like a plague. It came with a force, unlike any other; like the cancer that slowly kills, or the flood waters of a swollen river; there was no stopping them. The Warrior did not flinch or falter, because she knew that to do so would be the thing that could bring her down.

Then came the moment she had been waiting for; she glimpsed a way through the army's ranks to their king - if she could get to him, the army would retreat. So, without thought for her own safety, she ran forward into the midst of the fighting and before she could even consciously recognise what had happened, the King lay dead at her feet. She had defeated this dis-ease that had come to enslave her people and steal the land she knew as home.

As they retreated, she was swept away with her foe and eventually held as their prisoner. Although she had managed to save her people, she was to be put to death by those she had defeated. She did not care; for whilst death was frightening, she knew that she would be reunited with her beloved and that was the thing that made her tattered heart beat with joy.

As her captors scouted for a suitable place to execute her, they came across an old Alder tree, on a mount; the very tree where the Warrior and her love had spent some many long hours.

They tossed a rope over the lowest branch of the tree and formed a makeshift noose. The Warrior watched calmly as they prepared to take her life and although she knew not what to expect, she stood firm and looked blankly into nothingness. It seemed like hours before the small group placed the rope over her head and tightened it about her neck.

She closed her eyes and held the image of her love as clearly as she could, for his love was all that mattered now...

The Warrior Mystic faces the choices that are more challenging to make than any other - and they do so, because they have the strength to commit to their decisions. The Warrior as an individual acts as guardian to the whole being and will often be the aspect of the self that knowingly steps into the perspective of death, trusting they are reborn.

This does not mean the Warrior is selfless or comes to conclusions looking solely at the needs of others; it is merely this Mystic's ability to be strong in the face of adversity, so that they can attain greater levels of expansion. Just as a single cell will sacrifice itself for the survival of the body, the Warrior stands courageous in any situation.

When a cell dies, it does so in ecstasy - saturated in chemicals of euphoria. When the Warrior sacrifices themselves to release some dis-ease or trauma, they are immediately rediscovered at further level of expansion - for the Warrior is not separate or isolated; they are part of a much greater whole.

In other words, when you overcome a trauma or limitation whilst working with the Warrior, the Mystic will often become disconnected (as a facet of your emotional self that is no longer needed to exist in your awareness).

However, as you heal, you expand and therefore, reconnect to the Warrior once more, except on this occasion, the connection is at a greater layer of expansion

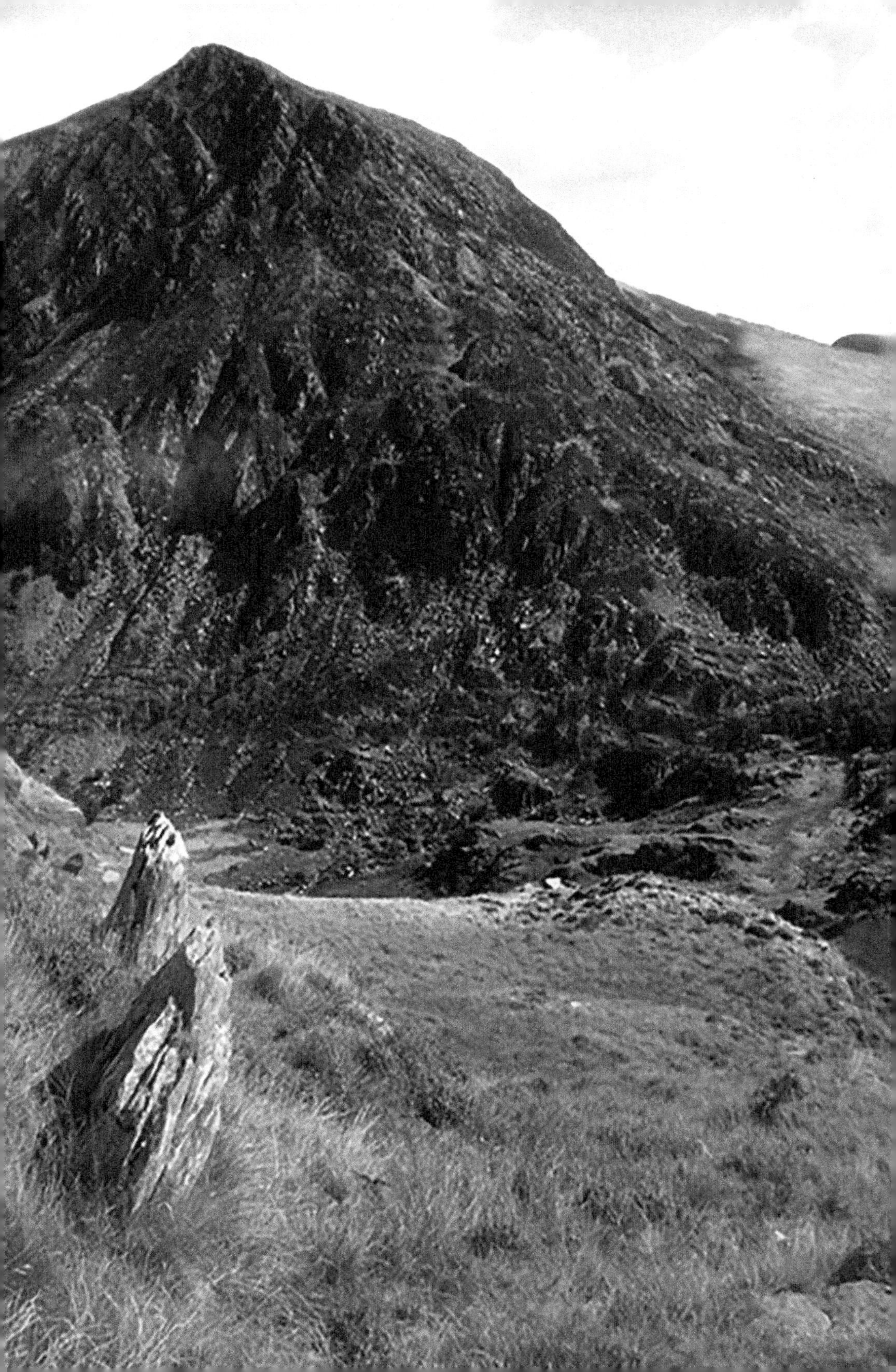

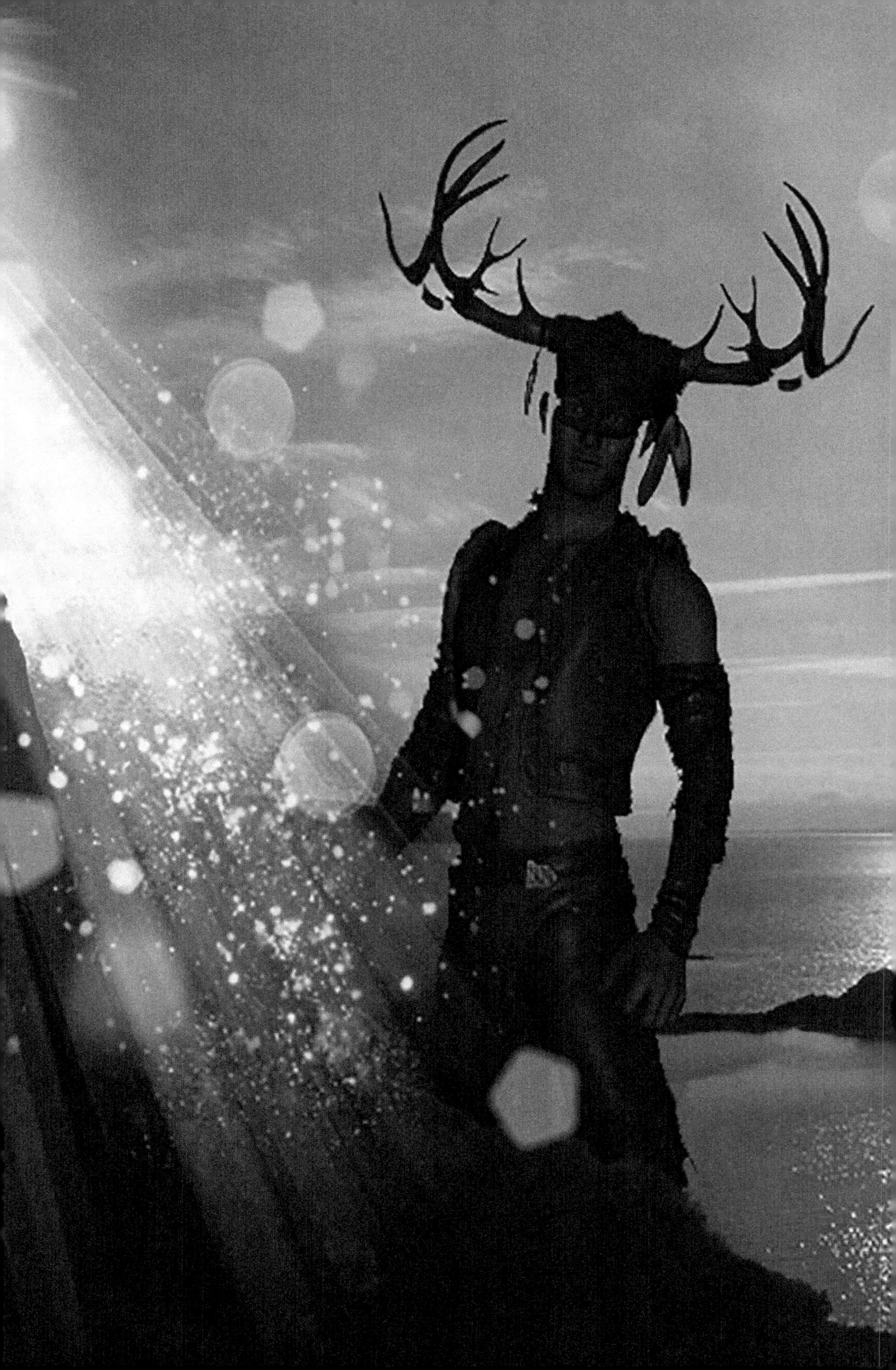

The Alchemist Mystic

The Alchemist made his way up the mound, towards the gnarled tree, admiring the ancient beauty of one so long-lived and full of wisdom. This old friend held many secrets, whispered by lost voices; he had eased the aching of many-a-heart that had long since stopped beating.

He approach the wrinkled, clay-coloured trunk which looked more stone than wood. The Alchemist reached out and touched the dry bark that turned to powder at his touch. With a long, deep inhalation, the man listened in the Fearn perspective and smiled a bittersweet smile as he realised the tree was dying.

"Old friend!" The Alchemist whispered. "How is it that you could live so much longer than all your fellow trees?"

The old Alder pondered this for a moment and then replied in his gravelly, booming voice that now held more gravel than boom.

"There are many secrets to be heard - some might say too many - and much pain to wash away. I have lived so long, not for the want of these things, but for a single hope... the hope that a little of that pain may be healed."

"Maybe I can help?" Asked the Alchemist earnestly.

"Alas," replied the tree. "I cannot tell you of the pain, for this would mean that I have betrayed a trust."

"Well, I could teach you how to create the situation where pain can be healed! I could show you the ways of the Alchemist!"

The tree waited a moment and then said, "If you were to share your wisdom with me, it would be just another secret and I am forbidden from using the secrets I know to help myself."

The Alchemist fell silent, for this was a paradox that required some thought - he could neither know the challenge, nor instruct the challenged. Any action seemed to go against the way of things, but he could not see his friend die without the granting of this simple wish—not one who had done so much for so many of his fellows.

This tree had seen so much of what is wrong with the world and just one simple act could make it better. A cuddle when one is feeling low, a bowl of freshly made soup when in the midst of the flu, a kiss from a sweetheart at the end of a long-lived life.

The Alchemist felt tears well up in his eyes. He knew that time was short and he must act fast before the tree slipped into unconsciousness. You see, for a tree who is dying of old age, the process is a slow one—it can sometimes take a whole summer and autumn, before the tree slips into winter's arms, never to wake again. Yet, as summer was past, the man knew that each day the Keeper of Secrets would fade from the physical world and not be able to recognise any action the Alchemist took.

"Allow your hope to carry you one day more, my friend!" The Alchemist murmured to the trunk, holding his lips close to the bark, so as not even the breeze could hear. "I shall return with the answer..."

And with that, the Alchemist left the tree on the mound; this confidant, this hero of so many that had fallen into disregard and was now noticed by so few. The man knew that he would find an answer to this conundrum, for this is the art of the Alchemist; the solver of puzzles and master of riddles.

The Alchemist is the manifester, the dream maker and granter of wishes. Yet, she is more than an intangible creature that plucks a whimsy from the air and waves a magic wand. Her methods are much more powerful, for she is logic and thought and creation through the art of definition.

The Alchemist will make the time to define each element of a detailed goal before directing her focus towards energetic creation. As such, an elaborate receptacle is formed - one that can contain all the power it needs to reach fruition in the physical world.

The Alchemist acts as a catalyst for synthesis (the coming together of many entities) and diversity (the splitting into separate entities). She weaves the magic that brings wholeness through the art of amalgamation or by the definition of individual identity.

The mentor and 'coach' of Celtic Reiki, the Alchemist is the most cerebral of the Mystics; focusing on the mind and expression in the external world via writing, print, and artistry. This Mystic will enable you to catch the fleeting moment in a well-structured definition that really personifies the core of your (or your clients') goals. As the 'thinker', the Alchemist also acts as a bridge between the spiritual and the emotional, enabling us to get the most deeply-felt experience of Celtic Reiki, whilst retaining the ability to communicate our experiences to others.

The Alchemist is also a problem-solver and master of riddles; for they think differently to others - see patterns, themes, and codes, where others see nothing but random nonsense. This ability is valuable in manifestation and goal-attainment, but also in treatments and master practices.

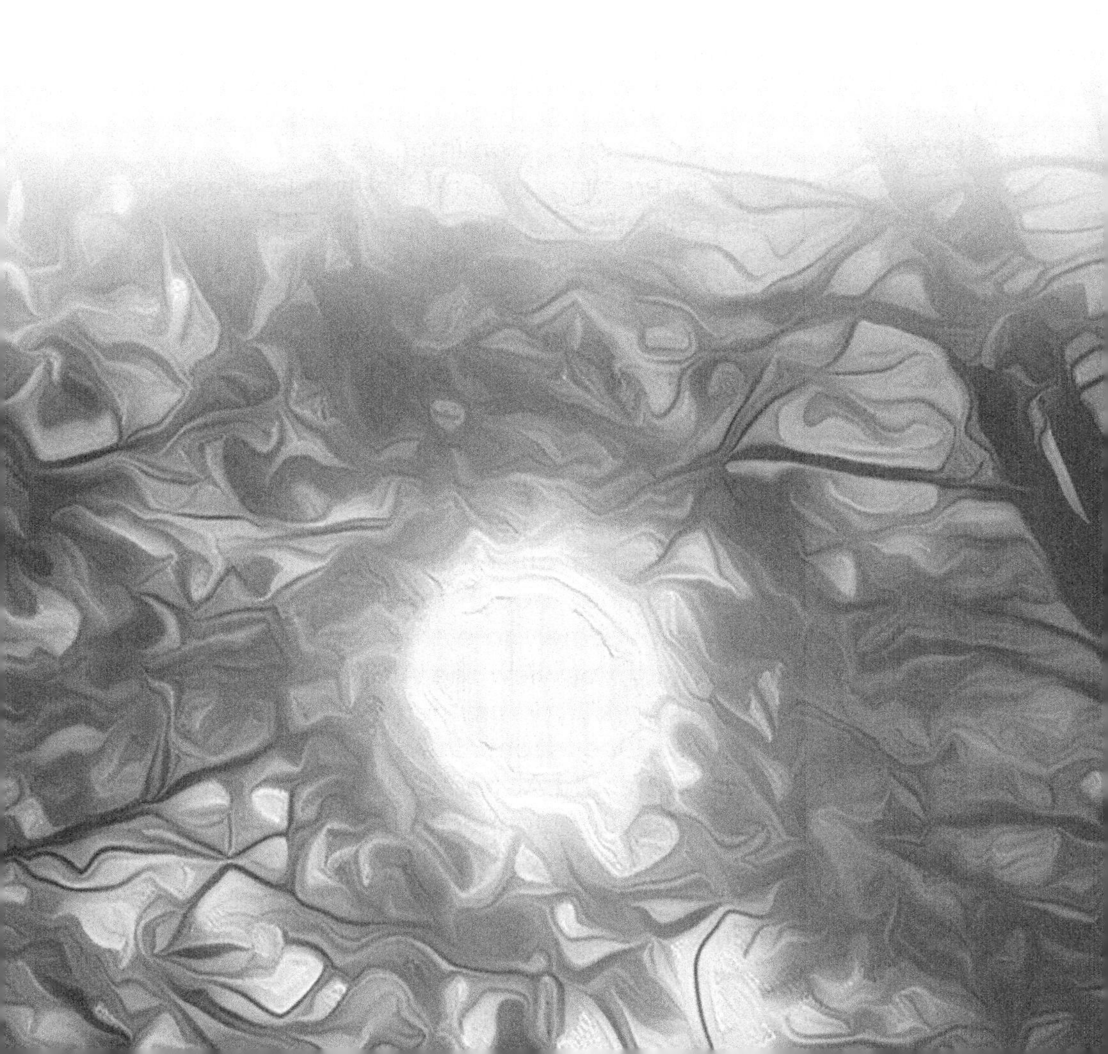

Connecting to the Alchemist

The Alchemist is the most cerebral of all the Mystics. Their focus being centred on the internal monologue, description and definition. The Alchemist relies on creating parameters to work with and as such, is the intellect to the Warrior's heart and Wise One's spirit.

Creating a connection to the Alchemist is far more about defining and being defined than either sensation or ritual. Conversely, the need to write (or present definitions in some more permanent way) is rather 'clunky' and could be inappropriate at times, so we tend to compromise a little, by creating a definition internally and then working within this definition through action and intent.

This means the techniques of the Alchemist are most similar in style to the Wise One, however, whereas the Wise One Mystic acts in faith, trust, and belief in a higher intelligence, the Alchemist's goals are expression through action, proactive use of knowledge and belief in one's own intelligence.

There is an interesting dynamic between these two mystics that, when connected to in a contractive manner, can lead to the Wise One's perspective of their counterpart as being calculating, scientific, and too sceptical.

Conversely, the Alchemist could view the Wise One as 'fluffy', ungrounded and flaky. This is an extremely important aspect of the discussion to highlight here, because it offers us an insight into occasions when we are causing the Mystics to contract to our perspective, rather than expanding to theirs.

The Alchemist is an integral aspect of Celtic Reiki, yet they are often dismissed in favour of the 'easier options'. The Alchemist can be challenging, though this is because we grow through challenge; we become more than we ever could be by taking the easy path. If you view the Alchemist methods to be too much like 'hard work', you are definitely in contraction. Alternatively, if the Wise One, seems insipid, or too 'airy-fairy', you are working in a contracted Alchemist state.

So, in the following connection method, you are presented with a choice—you can define your technique in writing or simply construct it 'internally'—either way is equally valid some of the time. The choice is dependent on the degree of physicality you want to offer your connection (and other techniques). There will be times when you want to be more fluid in your creation of the connection and other times, when you know that writing is an essential element in giving the connection 'structure'.

Your challenge will be, to recognise when you are too eager to favour one method over the other, though this is the learning curve that will lead you to self-mastery and the autonomous skills required for Master Mystic connection.

Technique:

1. Begin by defining your connection to the Alchemist - this means, stating why you have chosen to connect to the Alchemist on this occasion, how this connection will work to achieve specific results, and what results you particularly require. Write these down, create a Tree Plan, or simply list them in your head, depending on your situation.

2. With your plan in place, shift towards your Core State and then state your plan, either through reading your written definition, explaining your Tree Plan, or going through each step in your mind's eye.

3. At each point of definition, be aware of what Core State images, themes, thoughts, etc. move closer and which recede from awareness. Look for the patterns in these changes - are there consistent ingressions or regressions? Do you contract in certain areas of definition and expand in others? Are there any critical thoughts, scepticism, or feelings of resistance? Monitor these and create further definitions to counteract any contractive elements of your plan.

4. With your 'statement of definitions' completed, locate the Alchemist Mystic as a faraway star that glows brighter or a different colour from anything else.

5. Move the star towards you, keeping all else at bay and paying attention to any other aspects of your surrounding environment that attempt to block you

or limit you in any way. It is important to focus only on the 'star' as soon as you become aware of these other aspects.

6. Finally, connect to the star and step into your Alchemist self. Perceive the world in as much sensory depth as you can; ensure that you experience and proactively recognise their thought processes as often as possible. Write these down if appropriate, and pay attention to how this Mystic differs from the others.

7. When you are ready to disconnect, simply thank the Alchemist and visualise yourself stepping from the mystic and into your usual waking consciousness.

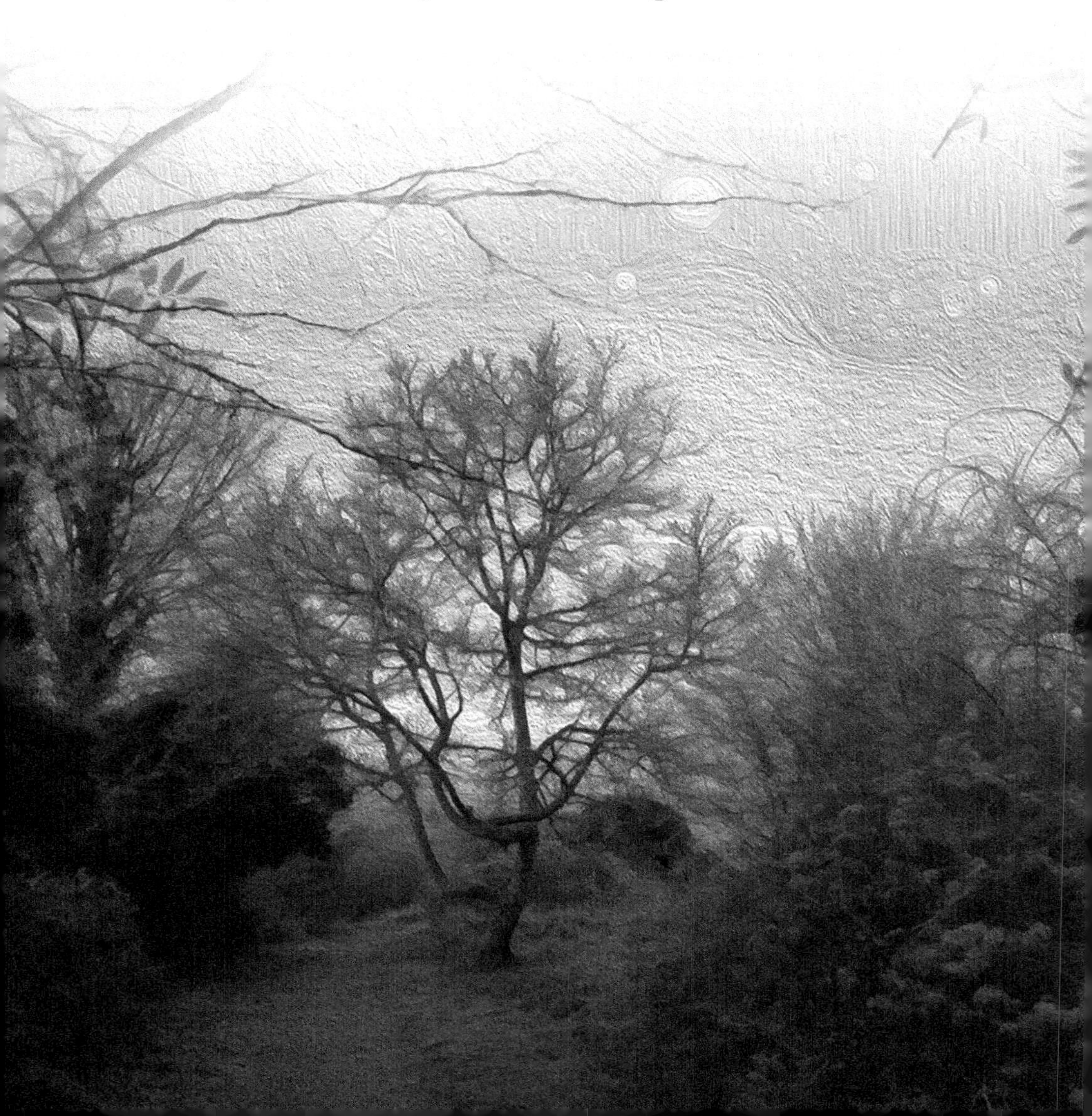

Realm Shifting with The Alchemist

This practice will help you to move between realms with ease and speed, making the transition between different dynamics and perspectives much easier to achieve during future exercises. A Celtic Reiki Realm Master can switch instantaneously from one realm to another.

The profound nature of the realms and how each realm affects you specifically, may mean that issues and dis-ease, and to a certain extent, perspective, will alter how fully you grasp each realm. The more your perspective (and other factors) can transcend your personal perspective and head into Realm Mastery for each unique realm, the greater your range of abilities will expand.

The previous treatments can be completed whilst doing other activities, however, I would recommend this treatment is conducted either seated or lying down for the utmost benefit.

1. Sitting or lying down with your arms and legs uncrossed and in a comfortable position, with your back straight, take your attention to your breathing. Take several deep breaths into your lower back and abdomen, using the same style of slow, regular breath as you have done with the previous exercises.

2. With each exhalation, find yourself expanding and on every in-breath, 'fall' into yourself, similar in experience to entering the Core State.

3. Internally affirm that you are entering "Avatar State" and repeat the mantra "Alchemist", three times, or use your favoured trigger method.

4. Feel a shifting from 'you', to 'you as the Mystic, Alchemist'. Wait a while for this and then proceed.

5. Choose the first realm you want to work with—such as the Woodland Realm, for instance—and internally, ask the Alchemist to "shift to the (x) realm" (where (x) is the chosen realm). As you do this, be aware of any changes in perception and note any synaesthesia responses you sense—write these down after the

experience for greater integrity of the final results.

6. Once you have entered the realm, explicitly describe your experience to 'fine-tune' your perception of this particular realm.

7. Once you have discovered your optimum realm experience, state internally to the Alchemist Mystic that you want to go to the next realm (stating your second realm choice by name, for example, the Standing Stones).

8. As you shift, be absolutely aware of any sensations, synaesthetic reactions and notable experiences that you can use to recreate this transition at a later date.

9. Once you have completed this for all five realms, come back into your conscious awareness of your physical environment and, when you are fully awake and focused, make detailed notes on your experiences.

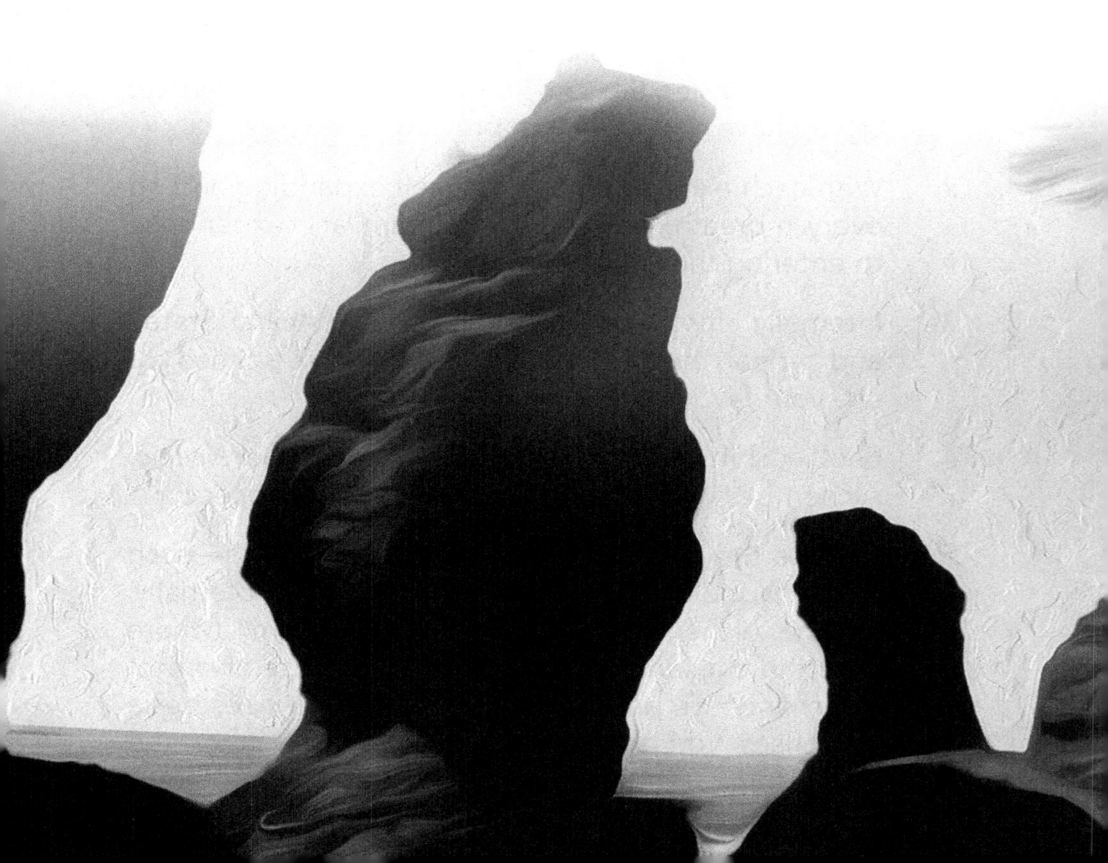

An Alternate Perspective

The Alchemist was wrapped in a profound introspection all the way back to his workshop; his magical place of spells and sorcery. How to make the dying wish of another come to fruition without knowing what they are wanting.

This was a paradox, for the art of the Alchemist requires focus and 'tight' definition to be most effective. For manifestation is both the creation of a receptacle (the 'shape' of what is desired) and the energy to 'fill it' (the magnetic force of attraction).

He sat at his desk and spent a while looking from the window, gazing past the Woodland Realm to the Furthest Mountains and beyond to the Cosmic Realm. His first thoughts of inspiration began to flicker into consciousness.

So he took a pen and wrote upon a piece of parchment—to fulfil a wanting that can be known. This was the trunk of his Tree-Plan and formed the basis for an elaborate design. It was the overriding outcome of this plan that very few people that are wanting, actually know what they want. They may have vague ideas, concepts, a focus on one thing when they actually yearn for something else—and most of all, the realisation that most people seek happiness; yet become side-tracked by the things they believe will make them happy.

If he could help manifest for others who knew very little of what they wanted, assisting the Alder would be simple. All he needed do was create a plan that detailed the end result of the Alder's experience, without ever mentioning how this would come about.

The Alchemist's skills in manifestation and intellectual development would activate the dynamic of attraction, the completion of which was a question of trust - trusting the Alder and the Universe to bring the perfect outcome into being. With that, he began to plan, to list the different parameters of his goal, and to focus on what he wanted to achieve for the Alder before the night came and the next adventure took him beyond this world.

Thought and careful planning are the tools of the Alchemist Mystic, for she details each step of the path and every piece of scenery along the way. The more definition she can give to any ritual contraction, will shift the focus from not having to having, wanting to realising that is it already ours. For the person that desires something they have not 'got', simply hasn't recognised the existence of the thing they want.

We live in the moment of now. If we imagine something that will be, counteracting that thought with 'soon but not yet', we are not bringing that thing into the now - the only place we ever consciously experience life. If we understand that the object or state of our wanting already exists for us, we begin searching for realisation of 'where' it is in our awareness. As we do this, we engage attraction and orientate towards the results we want.

The Alchemist Mystic knows this and sets about combining definition and attractive force. Synthesising desires from thought constructs and 'memes'. The Alchemical arts are about defining what is not yet recognised as physical. Everything you perceive was once a concept, a thought - one that has been refined and finely-tuned into reality.

From the architectural plans of a skyscraper and the blueprints for an aircraft, to the notes of a concerto, a painting, or a life lived with passion - all these were once thoughts, ideas, images in a person's head; energy that now exists in the solid world.

Though the Alchemist knows the philosophy of creation goes much deeper; for we literally think our world into being. From other people, to grains of sand, the sky, the trees, the stars, and the oceans—we believe them into reality, just as they perceive us into consciousness.

Perception and thought, interacting into a physical world, formed of infinite perspectives, infinite definitions. Some complement, others contrast, some even conflict, for conflict is the illusion that gives everything balance. Every edge is really two edges combined into the illusion of being one.

MANIFESTATION METHODS OF THE ALCHEMIST

THE COMPASS, THE MIST, AND THE CHALICE

In this manifestation method, we encounter three types of result—the goal, the desire and the hope. These are represented by the Compass, the Mist and the Chalice, which in turn, symbolise the focused direction of goals, the intangible, ethereal qualities of desires and undefined ambiguity of the relationship between the chalice and the liquid within.

Goals are well-defined, detailed statements of intent that focus the conscious mind towards the attainment of some state, situation or 'thing'. Goals are laid out in such a way that every aspect has been considered and the Alchemist has a very clear understanding of the results.

Desires are often feeling-based, with only vague or cursory definitions. Often a person will desire a 'thing' without knowing what exactly that 'thing' is, or why they want it. With desire can come frustration and longing, which actively repel the desire from ever being recognised.

Hopes are similar to desires, except they are more cerebrally-orientated and they have the potential for greater definition - hopes can be like an empty cup, water without anything to hold it in, or the water contained within a receptacle. With hopes, we realise the need for extensive definition (the chalice) and the magnetic force of manifestation (the water).

Using this technique, we use a compass to navigate through the mist and finish with a well defined hope - this creates a tangible sense of what is wanted - this is then shifted to, rather than 'created'. The idea of us possessing what we want, but simply not recognising it in the current moment is at the heart of this method and gives us the opportunity to locate the things we want, instead of grasping for them in the dark.

Technique:

1. Before you begin with any 'energy work', create a written plan, or Tree Plan defining the 'compass'. To be most effective, list 45 elements that describe this

goal; so if it is a new home, what type of windows will it have? What colour is the front door? And so on. When conducting this technique, a graphical representation is often easier to use, but if your prefer to write your list, have a good sense of what each thing looks, sounds and feels like.

2. Once this is completed, initiate your Core State, using your preferred method of breathing, visualisation and sensation.

3. In Core State, experience each point on your plan as a 'screen' around you. Some will be nearer than others, some distant and blurry. As you pinpoint each screen, the mist of desire will cover some of the screen, obscuring them completely or at the very least making them a challenge to see clearly.

4. With this image in your mind's eye, now visualise a chalice in front of you - it is empty. Describe what appears, using words and sensory experience to really clarify the chalice.

5. Move all the screens you can see clearly towards the chalice and see each one connect to it, becoming a gemstone on the outside edge.

6. Next, pull the mist into the chalice and see it becoming water. As each screen is revealed from behind the mist, bring it towards the chalice and create another gemstone.

7. Continue this process until the chalice is completely encrusted with jewels and full to the brim with water.

8. Centre yourself and then drink from the chalice. As you gulp thirstily, a distant screen appears, resembling a star. You move this towards you until you can clearly see the manifested result playing on the screen.

9. Finally step into the screen and come fully back into the room. Make notes about your experience.

THE GROVE OF CREATION

With this technique, you can conduct the processes and visualisations both for self-treatment, or when treating others. The only difference being that your client may possibly be in the room with you when you conduct the latter.

It is purely an individual choice, but you may like to involve your client consciously, by walking them through the visualisations.

One thing you may notice in the method laid out below is the lack of prescription (which essences to use), this is because the true meaning of manifestation is to state what you want and then heal the different aspects of yourself that are stopping you from obtaining that goal. There really is no difference between healing and manifestation! Therefore, the essences you use are down to what you intuit you should use and how you think they should be placed rather than using 'this tree' for 'that purpose'.

To help you with this, we work with two tree guides: The Lord of Thorns and Sanctuary Oak. They will offer a sacred space to conduct the manifestation treatment and help you intuit which essences to use and when.

Technique:

1. Prepare yourself for the treatment by centring yourself, closing your eyes, focusing on your breathing.
2. Shift into Core State and connect to the Alchemist Mystic.
3. Now ask the Lord of Thorns and Sanctuary Oak to be with you.
4. Standing at your client's head area, stand with your back straight, feet firmly on the floor and knees slightly bent. Make a head connection by placing your hands on or over your client's temples and await a good sense of connection between you.
5. Now state the intent of the manifestation treatment, i.e., what it is that you or your client wishes to manifest. Then trigger the essence(s) you feel necessary; in the

original version of Celtic Reiki, this would primarily be Nuin.

6. Now visualise a sacred grove in front of you, seeing two large trees creating a gateway – let the images flow and do not try to force them. If you find it easier to create a sense of imagery by hearing or feeling, listen to the sound of the wind in the leaves or explore the trunks of the trees with your internal senses, imagining what they would feel like to the touch. It is important to remember, energetically you are actually in the grove and that it is not imagined!

7. Now, with this scene firmly in your mind, place your hands on your lap for self treatment or on your client's shoulders. Then, in your mind's eye, see yourself leading them through the 'gateway trees' and into a sacred sanctuary, deep in the heart of the grove.

8. In this sacred space are a group of trees that form a circle all around you – there can be as many or a little as you like, although 12 is a good number as you can base the layout on the face of a clock. Each tree should be relevant to your purpose and you can have many trees of one species if you wish. You may find that you do not recognise what some of the trees are, or you may want to use a tree that you have not physically encountered before, so cannot visualise it accurately – neither of these considerations matter, as the exercise will work regardless.

9. In the centre of the circle, see the Lord of Thorns—a regal holly tree, and The Sanctuary Oak – a strong and powerful Oak tree with his limbs outstretched to nurture. Keep your assertion of energy strong and guide your client towards the Holly and Oak, stating the intent for this treatment.

10. Now all the trees begin to glow with light, getting brighter and brighter as the treatment is conducted, the light gets so bright in fact, that you feel waves of energy projected towards you from every tree. Breathe in this energy and project it through your client using

your out-breath to help focus the Celtic Reiki and your manifestation intent.

11. Now you may either stay at the client's head/shoulder area, or move around them, depending on what your preference is. All the time, try to maintain the image of the grove in your mind, until your subject starts to glow with the energy too.

12. At the end of the treatment (which can last between thirty minutes and an hour depending on the time you have set aside), thank the trees in turn and the Alchemist. Then lead your subject back through the gateway and then close down in whatever way you intuit.

13. Ask your client to return to the room, check that they are fully-awake, and offer them a glass of water.

You can also adapt this treatment to work as a self-treatment by imagining yourself on the treatment couch and conducting the routine with the proviso that you receive the treatment when you lay on the couch—then lay down on the couch for an hour to reconnect with the energy. I like to view this technique as reflecting two parts of the self—the Alchemist who conducts the treatment and the Client who calibrates to it.

You can also conduct a self-treatment by simply sitting in a chair and running through the meditation for yourself, by yourself.

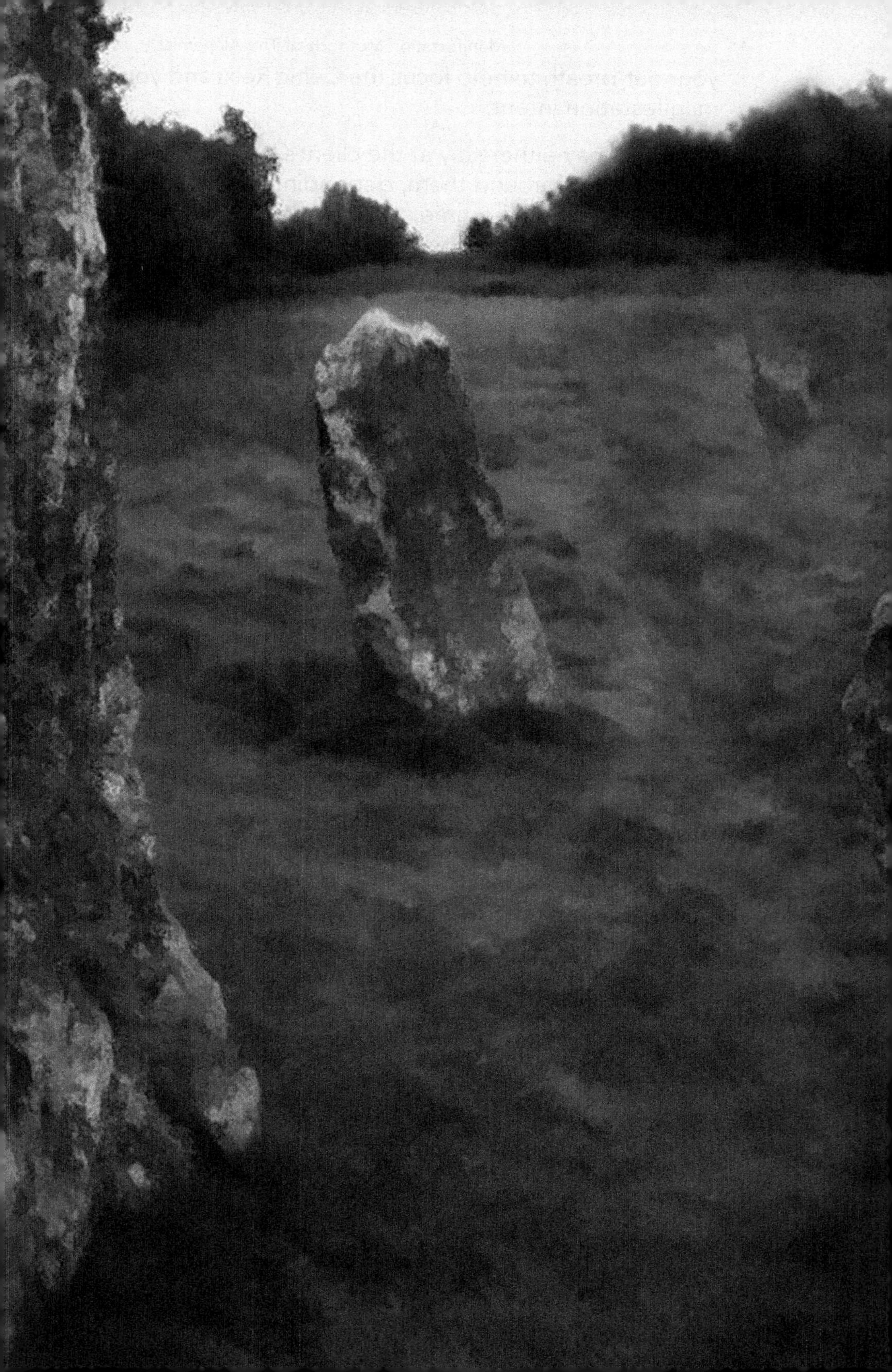

The Alchemy of Celtic Reiki

Alchemical Synthesis & Diversity

The two final dynamics of the Alchemist that are of relevance here, are those of synthesis and diversity—we bring elements together and we act as a catalyst for separation. Both have an equal value to the art of manifestation and the greater purpose of the Alchemical perspective.

There are times when we require the connection of situations, perspectives, dynamics, or other elements - such as the combination of essences, or the joining of Core State to desired outcome.

There are also occasions when we require diversity, such as when separating a person from their limiting beliefs, or when we want the finer nuances of an essence that can be split into 'individual' layers or sources.

The scope of both these methods is so wide ranging in effect that it is very much down to the individual Alchemist and contexts they encounter, as to how the following are used. It is, therefore, vital for you to recognise that these techniques form dynamics, which can then be applied to various scenarios, rather than techniques that cause a specific result.

Imagine you have two situations: in one you want to bring elements together and in the other, separate them. In the former—Alchemic Synthesis—you are creating a perspective of flour and water. Here the elements will clump together, forming something more 'solid' in nature. Alternatively, the Alchemic Diversity will act like the perspective of oil and water - completely diverging into their own 'place'.

Now compare the different qualities a person needs to succeed as grains of flour and their limiting beliefs as oil. By adding the same thing, you get different results.

The essential factor is that each aspect is defined differently and that the technique is used separately for the different dynamics - add water to flour and oil combined, and you get a foul-tasting cake!

Technique:

1. Decide on the results of this technique, before conducting the following routine. In other words, do you require synthesis or diversity? This is like saying "this is flour" or "this is oil", where the technique itself is the water. Jot down what it is you want to bring together or pull apart and list each aspect of this. For instance: what are the qualities you wish to combine? What do you want to separate from what?

2. Once you have chosen your outcome, enter your Core State, using your preferred method and shift to the perspective of the Alchemist Mystic.

3. Once in your centred, non-reactive place, state internally either 'diversity' or 'synthesis' three times and then continue with the following steps in an identical way for either outcome.

4. See the result in front of you to the left and the action of 'alchemy' ahead and to the right. There is no need to state which form of alchemy you require - the 'action' is enough.

5. Trigger your preferred manifestation essence - this could be Nuin, Ur, Gold, etc. And experience the essence bursting from within the action (right hand side), as if being created from within the action.

6. The next stage of the process is to bring the result and the action together, slowly and steadily. Watch the two facets of the process converge and then experience the 'reaction' through visualisation, sensation or synaesthesia. This will be very different on each occasion.

7. When the process is complete, return to waking consciousness and make notes on what occurred.

The Path to Mastery... Integrating the Three Mystics

Mastery of any art is not something that can be truly achieved through the study of a course or workshop - even though these are essential as a foundation. A certificate does not make the Master and there is no point at which you become a Master. The thing is that we are always the Adventurer, exploring, learning, growing. We are the Wise One, the Warrior and the Alchemist; healing, becoming more confident in our abilities, and manifesting with ever-increasing success.

Yet, it is none of these things that make us a Master of Celtic Reiki; it is our conduct in the experiencing of these things that form our Mastery. A person can call themselves a Master and yet behave in an egocentric, dominating, or uncaring way, without consideration for others. The Apprentice who acts with foresight, compassion and joy has a greater Mastery than any person with the title, but none of the qualities.

I was the first Celtic Reiki Master and have been blessed by that title for well over a decade, however, there are times when I have not acted with real mastery. On those days, I was not a Celtic Reiki Master. Conversely, when I have earned my title, through the guidance or support of another, through interaction with the trees, or by noticing something within myself that helps me grow or contribute to the Earth in some way, I feel like a Master.

So, we now embark on the next segment of the journey - to discover the nature of the Master Mystic and the understanding that we do not become a Master and stop being an Apprentice. We spend each moment striving for mastery and learning how to achieve that state as much as we can, each day.

We shall take our connections to the other Mystics and explore how each can guide us to something that is never taught, nor learned through repetition - it is a burst of light that each of us can be, if we decide to commit to being that light...

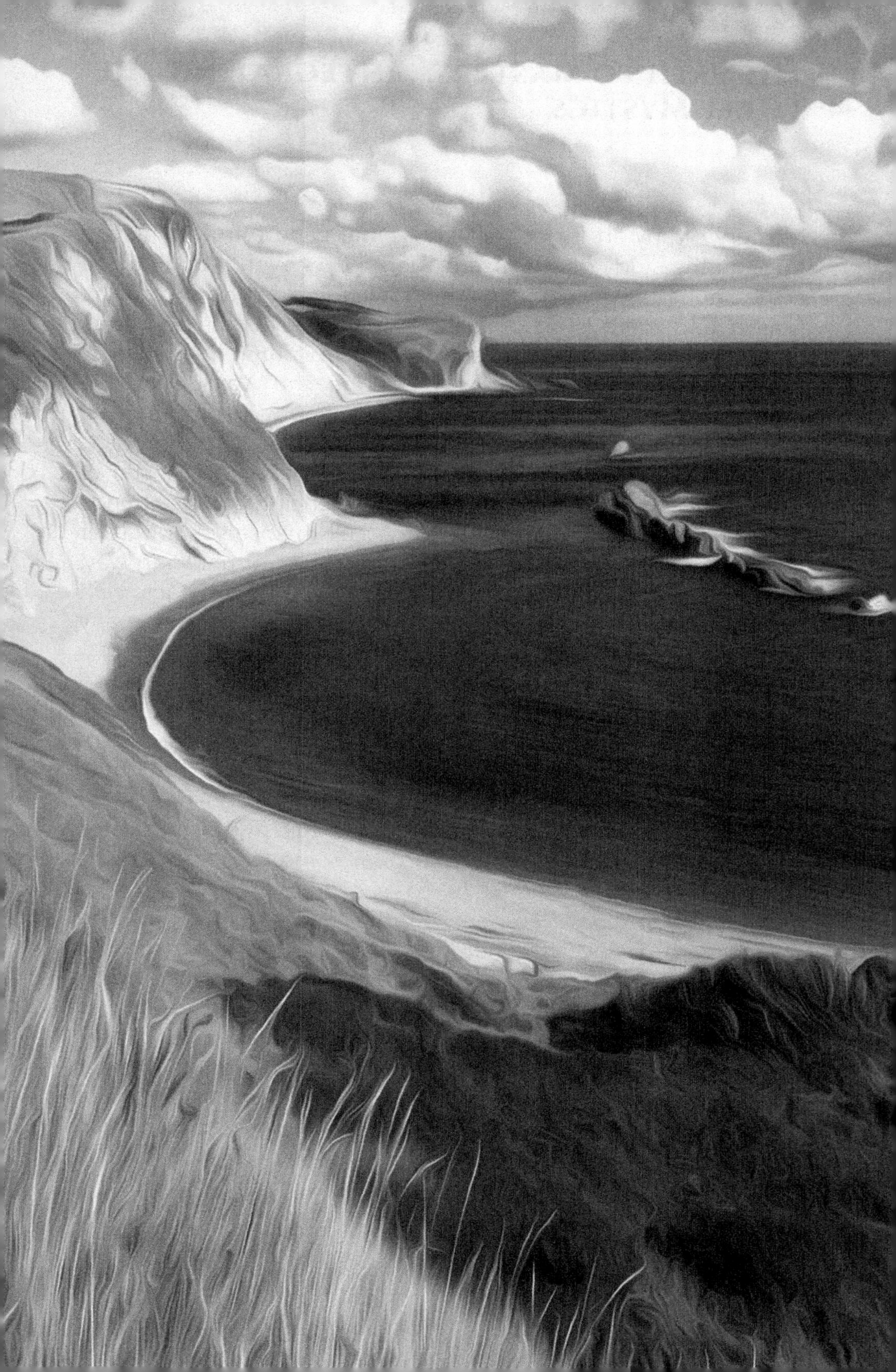

Three Paths into One...

The Alchemist drew back from the ancient Alder, overwhelmed by the joy that flooded from every inch of his being. If ever a tree was capable of a smile, this faltering, dying old hunk of wood, was so wrapped in the wide and upturned expression of rapture as to be like any child, caught up in the timeless moments of play.

As the Alder watched the two lovers embrace, he was whole; his life had meaning. Through all the hurt and despair he had listened to throughout his long life, the fact he now knew pain can be completely healed, and trauma, in a moment transcended, he would leave this physical world, without regret or a tear for those he had known as friends.

For if the Earth was able to find the time for such miracles, such incredible happiness, then he knew that we exist in a place where all pain and hardship is transcended. Problems stop being problems and whatever it is we grieve for and break our hearts over is merely a fleeting and finite thing.

The Alchemist stayed a while, as the grand Alder slipped into a peaceful slumber and retreated from the world for the last time...

They led the Warrior Queen towards the mound where the Keeper of Secrets reached up to the moon, almost as if praying for some other fate. That his branches be used by man to take a life and what's more, the life of a friend who was so precious and kind. He had known her, child and adult; he was her companion through pain and tribulation and now he was her executioner.

As they marched her towards death, to an unimaginable ending in a place that symbolised healing and the transcendence of pain, she did not fear. Her legs were strong and there was no sign of buckling as her knees supported her onwards. Even when they reached the canopy of the Alder's branches, she did not cry or plead or feel anything other than love.

For the Warrior is not of war, she is of kindness and strength. She fights for love and for those who cannot find their way when the night is at its darkest. She fixed her mind on the knowledge that all would be good with the world and with her.

She focused on the man she loved with all her heart. This man that came from so far away; the man she would never hold, whose face could not be touched, and of warmth she would never feel.

As the cold roughness of the rope wrapped around her neck, she took one last glimpse at the blue-tinged moon, before closing her eyes and returning her thoughts to him. Only him.

The man sat in his favourite chair, facing away from his death—wanting so much to hold on to life in these last few seconds of awareness. He heard a footfall on the carpet behind him and closed his eyes, weeping uncontrollably as each second seemed to reach out into the infinite and last forever.

He felt a hand on his shoulder, a strong and warm hand that he knew would be the last sensation he ever felt, and with a final, all-encompassing breath of air, of life, he died.

He felt himself standing. But how could this be, for he was dead? He had been so certain that hand was the hand of death that he was on his feet and turned around before he even thought about opening his eyes.

As he took the very first glimpse of his new life, he saw the shining beauty of his love, felt their warm embrace for the very first time and fell into their arms. His handsome knight in shining amour, his warrior, his soulmate. And with that, the man who was so irredeemably lost to the world and to love, was reborn.

The Warrior Queen stepped down from the noose, guided by some unseen guide, some faraway kindness, some alchemist of lives and love. And just as if he had always been there, she saw her love sitting before her in what seemed like a favourite chair. He was afraid, trembling in the wake of some unseen fear. So, walking up to him, she placed a loving hand on his shoulder and with the gentlest pressure of her fingers, guided him to stand, facing her.

Gradually, he opened his eyes and took a moment to adjust to the light, to her face. And as he gazed into her eyes, she knew that he did not look upon her as others had done. He did not see her, based on costume and role and all of the other petty labels humankind is so eager to give. He saw love; the same love as she. And with that, they fell into each others arms; their secrets intact, but no more pain; no more pain.

As the Alder drifted blissfully from life, he heard the Alchemist's voice whisper in the human tongue and felt the familiar Fearn translation accompanying him on his next adventurer...

"My dearest friend, I have one last secret for you to keep...

...A single act of kindness, no matter how seemingly insignificant, can wash away a lifetime of pain. For kindness is the last thing we know in life; it is the blanket that warms us as we tumble into the unknown. For kindness stems from love and love, as we all know, is the most powerful force in the Universe.

Love is beyond definition; more than faces and names - love knows no gender, no status, no dis-ease, no time, and no space. When we love somebody, truly love somebody, it does not matter whether they are man or woman, human or tree or puppy dog. Love is not decided on whether a person takes this action or complies with that demand; it just is.

Love can be felt so strongly that a person will choose the hardest road, each and every day so that they may love to the fullest. They are beaten, spat upon, turned away, hated, excluded, persecuted, put to death, and at every turn denied their natural rights of dignity, belonging and acceptance, all because of the slightest word, expression, assumption, or implicit value. Yet, when asked, they would make the same choices time and time again.

Love can seem strange and may even distort our perception of life and of others, yet all this fades into nothingness when we measure it against the ability of love to bring us together across unimaginable distances, regardless of faith, or race, or opinion.

Love pushes us past our fragile connection to the physical body; beyond a momentary life that seems so full of experience, yet is often missed when entangled in memories. Love wakes us up, causes our hearts to beat faster and our desire to be, stronger.

Love cannot be stopped, hindered, taken-away, or lost. It is intertwined with every piece of everything that exists, and yet, we cannot see it or touch it, except in the precious, fleeting moments we make for ourselves and for others. A glance, a touch, a gesture, a word, an act—just a small act of kindness."

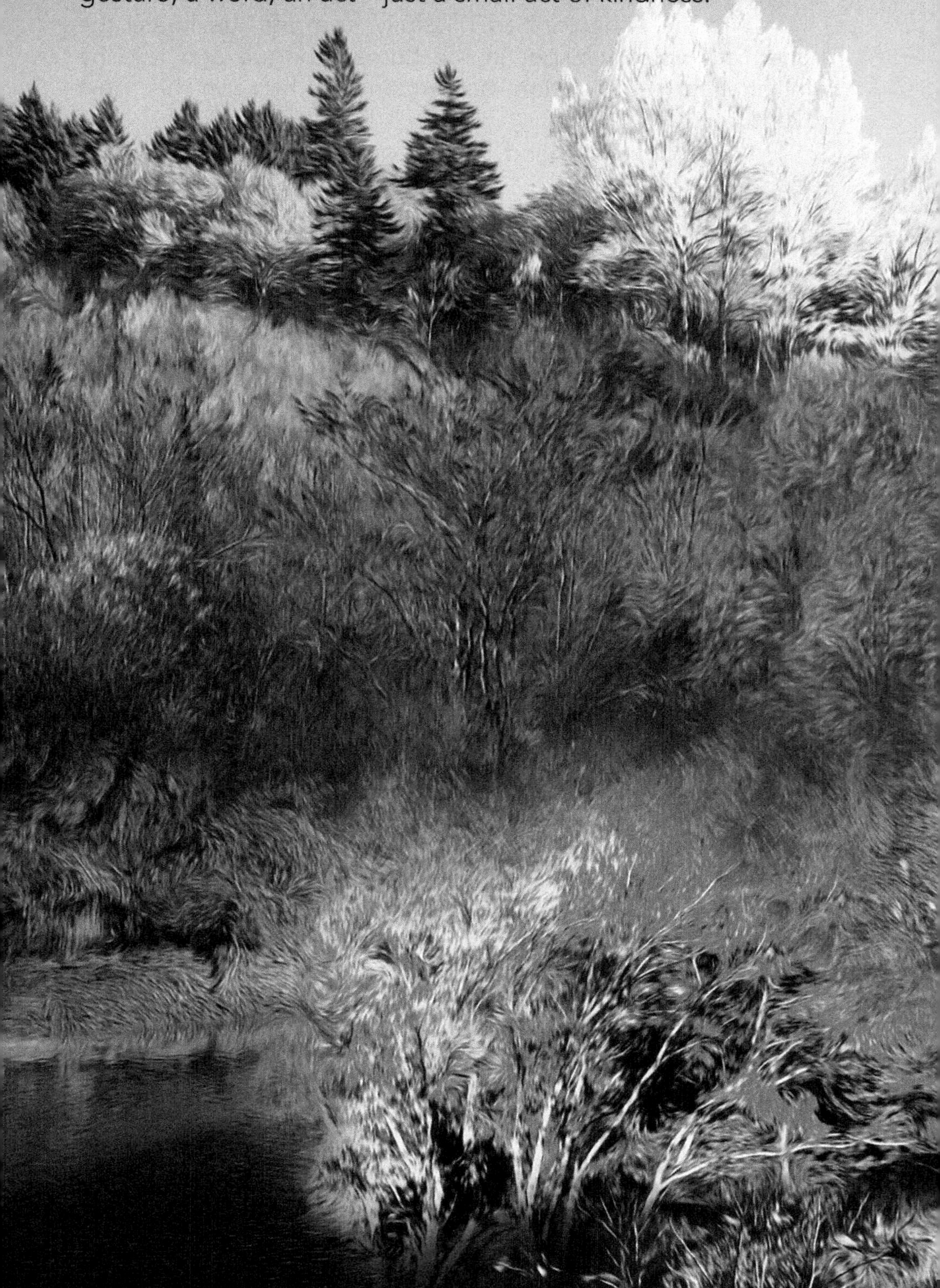

Other Celtic Reiki Books in the Home Experience:

This book is part of the Celtic Reiki Mastery Home Experience from mPowr—to enrol visit the Official Celtic Reiki Website at www.celtic-reiki.com.

The Adventurer's Guide

The Encyclopaedia of Celtic Reiki Essences

A Master's Companion

The Realm Master's Almanac

Realm Master: Secrets (The Sacred Wisdom of Celtic Reiki)

Discover the ***Bedtime Stories of the Woodland***, now available from mPowr Publishing: the enchanting tales from the Celtic Reiki Mastery Home Experience within a single VAEO. Read the stories, hear the narration*, and interact with the characters*. Experience the wonder of the Realms anew...

*when used in conjunction with your smart phone or camera-enabled tablet device

Audio Programmes from the Author:

Synaesthesia Symphony IV: The Chorus of Creativity

Synaesthesia Symphony V:The Harmonies of Health

The PsyQ Orientation

For further information about Celtic Reiki, The Celtic Reiki Mastery Home Experience, and vReiki Training please visit:

www.celtic-reiki.com
www.mpowrpublishing.com

Lightning Source UK Ltd.
Milton Keynes UK
UKOW06f1417121117
312604UK00004B/84/P

9 781907 282409